Kamasutra Sex

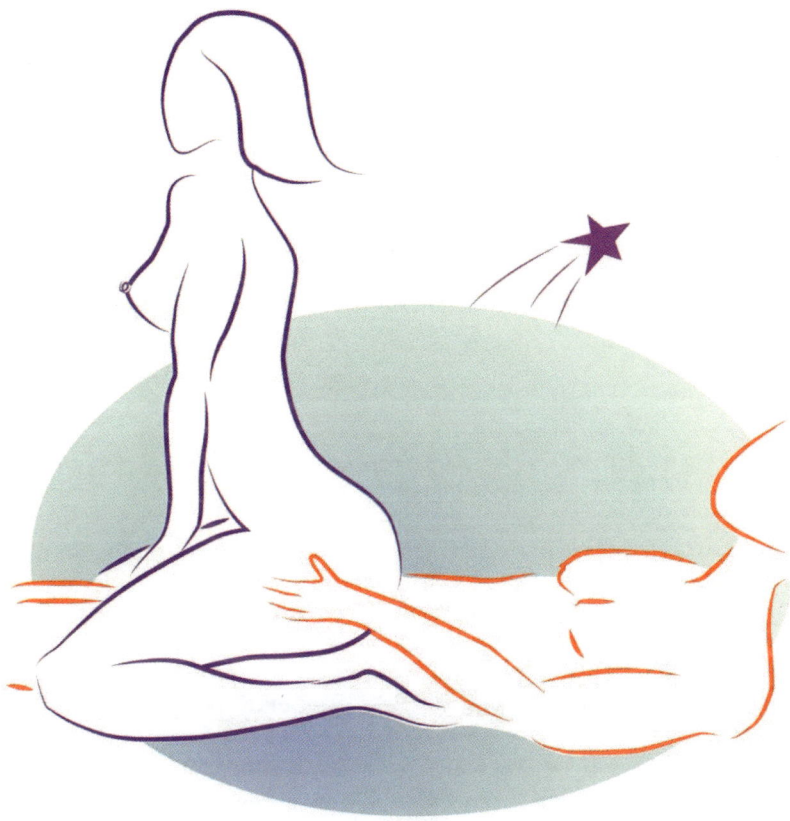

Over 50 Sex Positions

W T McCleat with Susan Florence

Copyright ©2013 SandSPublishing
Published by: SandSPublishing
First printed September 2013 - First Edition
ISBN-13: 978-1492771913 – Print Version
ISBN-10: 1492771910
Created & Printed in The United States of America, Distributed Worldwide.

Other Books by W.T. McCleat and Friends

Massage Erotica: Foreplay to Seduction
Cheating Romance of Wives, Husbands & Lovers
Divorced Women: Our Sexual Liberation & Discovery
Taboo Sex to Erotic Enlightenment (Midsummer's Night Taboo)
Betrayed by Love: Tangled Web of Lust and Desire
An Erotic Love Triangle: Tale of Erotic Romance
World War II Warplanes: The Iconic Warplanes of World War II
Vintage Cocktails Forgotten Cocktails & Timeless Drinks
Kamasutra Sex Positions: Sex Positions with Seductive Cocktails

Available on most fine on-line retailers and discounted on
SandSPublishing.com/wp-store W T McCleats publishing company

Your Kamasutra

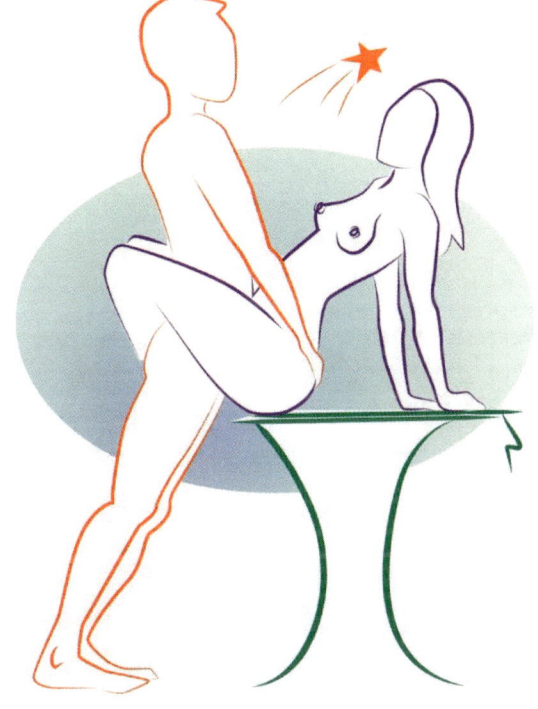

Your Party Your Way

Table of Content

Why Over 50's Kamasutra?

Over 50's Kamasutra is a guide for those of us who are not quite as flexible as we used to be, yet want the stimulation of trying new and unusual positions for sex to spice up our love life. I, W T McCleat and my partner, are both over the 50 mark by a few years. We found that our sex life was becoming monotonous yet our love was strong for each other. We devised a plan to systematically find different and fun sex positions that we could do easily without straining ourselves yet getting the erotic stimulation we both so desired.

After many months of practice we devised the 'Over 50's Kamasutra' guide for those of us that seek the fun of lovemaking. Not only was it fun to try these positions but it had many other benefits; enhanced love making, spiritual wellbeing, more flexibility over time, relaxed deep desire for each other and a removal of all inhibitions that we had inadvertently collected over the years.

In this guide we also added a few simple stretching exercises that quickly began to be the foreplay for some very intimate sex. These stretch positions helped us to become more flexible but added a spiritual essence to love making that we had never experienced before. The stretching of our bodies also helps to empty our minds of the daily clutter of thoughts leaving a purified sense of wellbeing with a deep down desire for each other. It was as if the some superior being was applauding our natural way of finding the hidden depths of each other's desires, wants and tenderness. This became the driving force that solidified our union into something far more physical than bodily union, the actual true mating of our minds which was by far the most intimate moments we have ever experienced from many of the Over 50's Kamasutra positions.

Over 50's Kamasutra will open up a complete new approach to foreplay and intense sexual and spiritual satisfaction. It is like a 'gateway drug' that is completely safe yet leads you to heights of sensual enlightenment. I and my partner believe that as we age our desire for spiritual influence becomes a strong force that needs to be released from our inner desires. We have found that the Over 50's Kamasutra positions allows the release of this energy which provides a true deep down desire to please and be pleased.

If you find that your lovemaking is beginning to get lack luster, yet you do still have deep desire for your partner then it is time to look through this guide and begin a journey of discovery. Our advice is to start slowly perhaps trying a few simple stretching exercises in front of each other preferably naked. This will be a huge stimulus especially as you find it fun and laughter will prevail which instantly breaks down any inhibitions. If you feel you need more sustenance to begin such a journey then try our book 'Kamasutra with a Twist: Sex Positions with Seductive Cocktails'. A small amount of such beverages will not only help reduce any inhibitions but taken at the right time will stimulate some of your bodies erogenous zones making for a more pleasurable and deep experience.

We also suggest some gentle stretch exercises to limber you up. Consider it foreplay, a simple yet erotic warm-up for things to come! So that you enjoy the Over 50s positions try these simple exercises that will limber you up. We suggest you do these in the nude to create anticipation and arousal. At the end of this book each warm-up position is explained in detail.

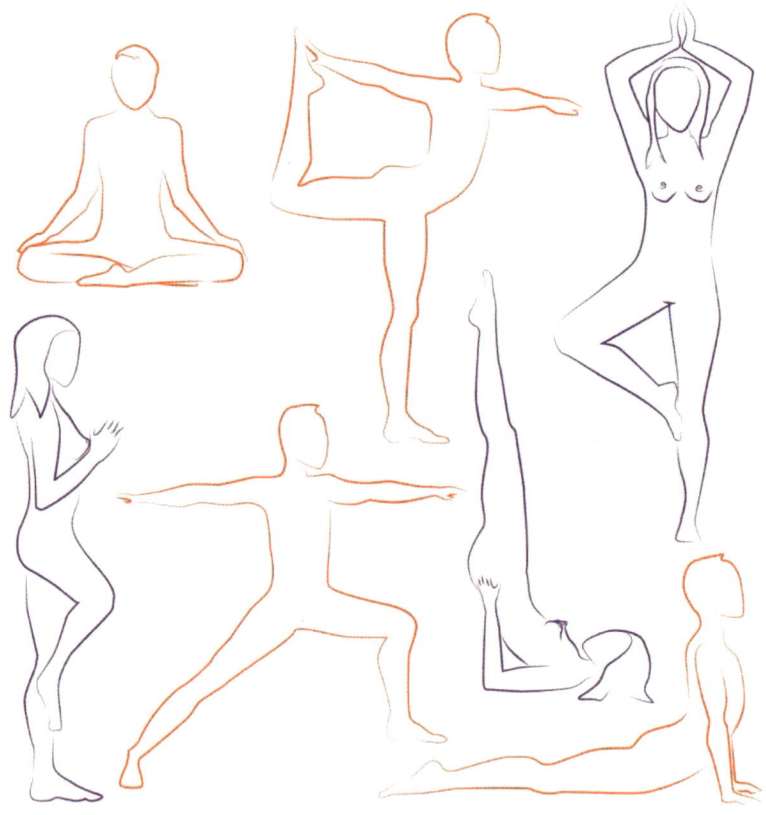

Read through his book but keep it close to your bed. Intimacy and desire should be your pleasures, don't wait; seek the true and satisfying depths of your physical and spiritual needs through the 'Over 50's Kamasutra'!

'Eye to Eye' Style

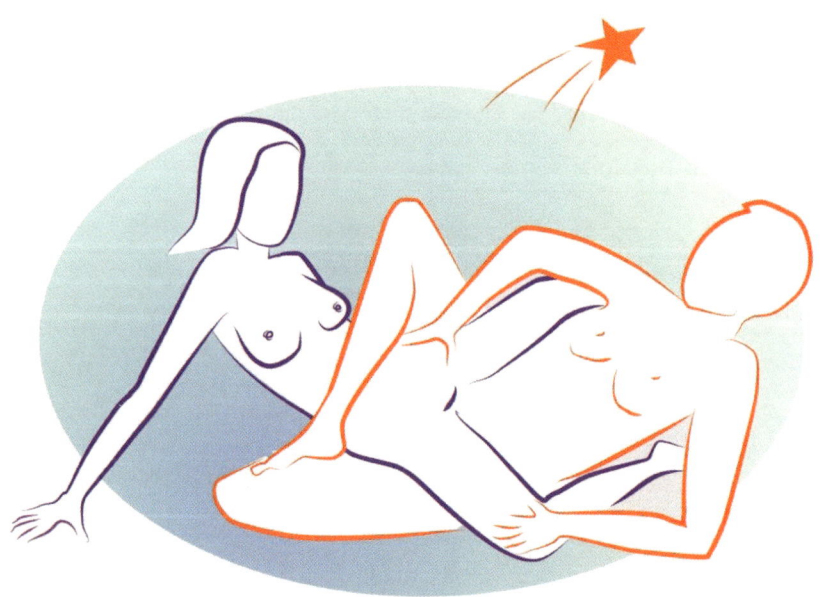

The 'Eye to Eye' position allows each partner to look at the pleasures they are giving to each other. It takes a deliberate effort to get into this very sensuous position. Both move to sit down opposite each other. She wraps her legs around him helping to guide him into her. Both can look into each other's eyes as they push to get deeper into her. He then wraps his one leg over her securing her in place. She will need to brace herself by her arms leaning back. He must be propped up on his elbow to provide leverage as he pushes in and out of her.

'Deep Probe'

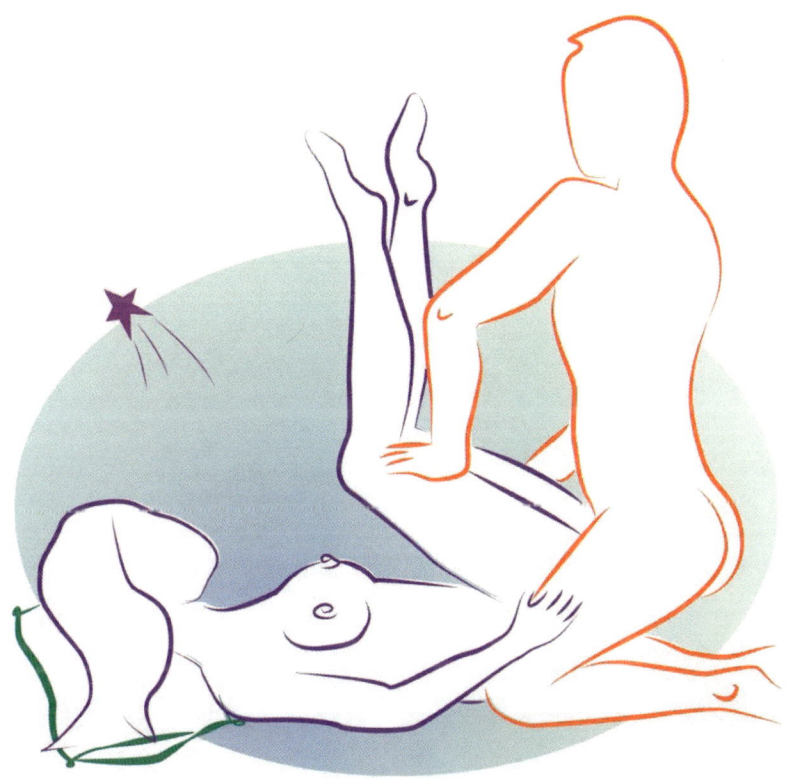

The 'Deep Probe' posture or alternatively described as *'Bottoms Up'* gives deep penetration but keeping your legs high overtime becomes a challenge. You may need to try this position often to build leg muscle!

She lies on her back pulling her knees up to her breasts reaching her feet toward the ceiling. At this point her hips should be off the bed. He kneels placing his thighs under her raised bottom allowing her to rest her bottom on him as he pushes himself into her. Once inside her he can change the angle of his strokes by using his free hand to push her legs further back pushing his thighs closer to support her more so she can enjoy the stroking without tensing her body until an orgasm occurs.

A pillow to prop her head up allows her to watch the action of his movements in and out providing her great sensual anticipation. A real turn on for her as this is a gentle relaxing position. Once mastered it is very satisfying for the woman because of the slow deep penetration.

'Sweetness' Position

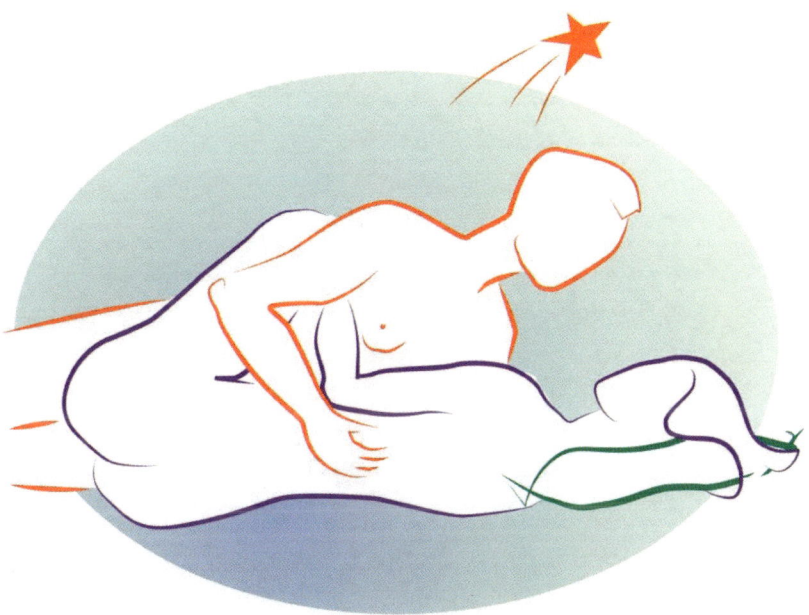

The 'Sweetness' is a fun position with the man sliding between her legs; she's lying on her side with her knees bent.

She encircles him with her legs and crosses her ankles behind his back, gripping him with her thighs. He thrusts in and out while her hands are free to caress his neck or nibble, his ear lobes and whisper to him exactly what she'd like him to do next.

Tempting 'Erotic Tilt'

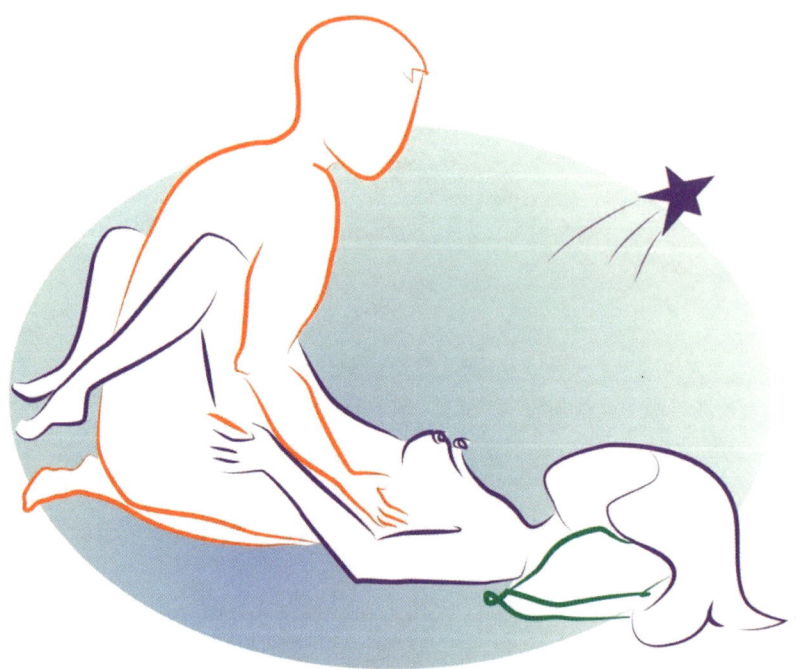

To achieve the 'Erotic Tilt' she lies on her back with open, outstretched legs. The man sits between her knees, facing her with legs straight out or folded under him.

He lifts her hips to aid penetration and at the same time he can lean down to kiss her belly providing he's flexible enough. Wonderfully romantic positions, allowing your partner to relax as you caress her breasts and stomach while you gently rock inside her. This is not a deep penetration position, but great for partners who prefer partial entry. Both can look lovingly into each other eyes as this act is performed. In cool climates it is ideal, as it maximizes the heat between bodies. For the guy the gentle movement will stimulate him plus the gently swaying of the female breasts is very sensual to watch.

'Fondling Rider' Rob Roy Style

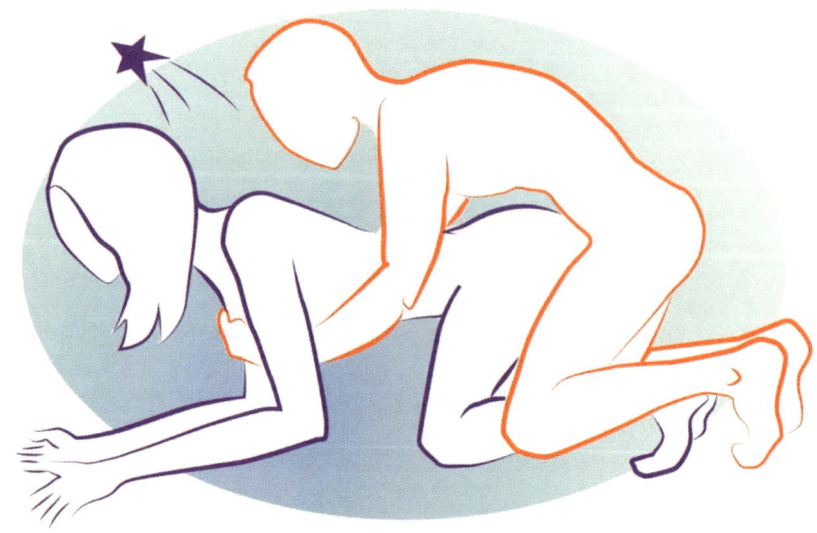

'Fondling Rider' is a variation on doggy style, a real backdoor intimate position where she's still on all fours but lowers herself onto her forearms and he penetrates her deep from behind as he reaches around to caress her breasts. Hold on to them firmly the going may get very bouncy and totally enjoyable for all!

View of the 'Magic Ride'

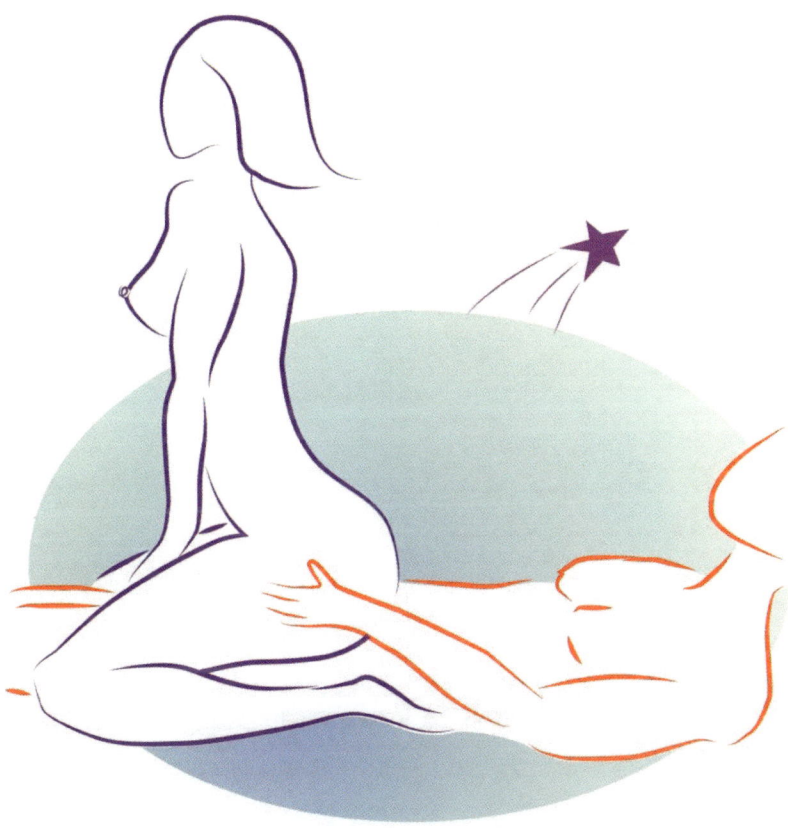

In the 'Magic Ride' posture, she kneels astride her partner but with her back to him as she leans forward to balance herself on his knees with her hands giving more balance or thrust, as needed.

He holds her waist and thrusts upwards, while she slides up and down on top of him with a spirited thrusting, providing a rhythmic view of her soft curvaceous bottom, very erotic indeed. Her hands are available to play with her partner's genitals as he stimulates her anal area and applies pressure strokes on her perineum. Oh my! Perhaps some gentle spanking will provide that little extra excitement and naughtiness. Very erogenous for the woman as she begins her ascent to climax. Very exciting for the guy as he watches her pulse on him. Don't be surprised if he plays with her anus. Pure unadulterated eroticism!

Incredible 'Table Wrap'

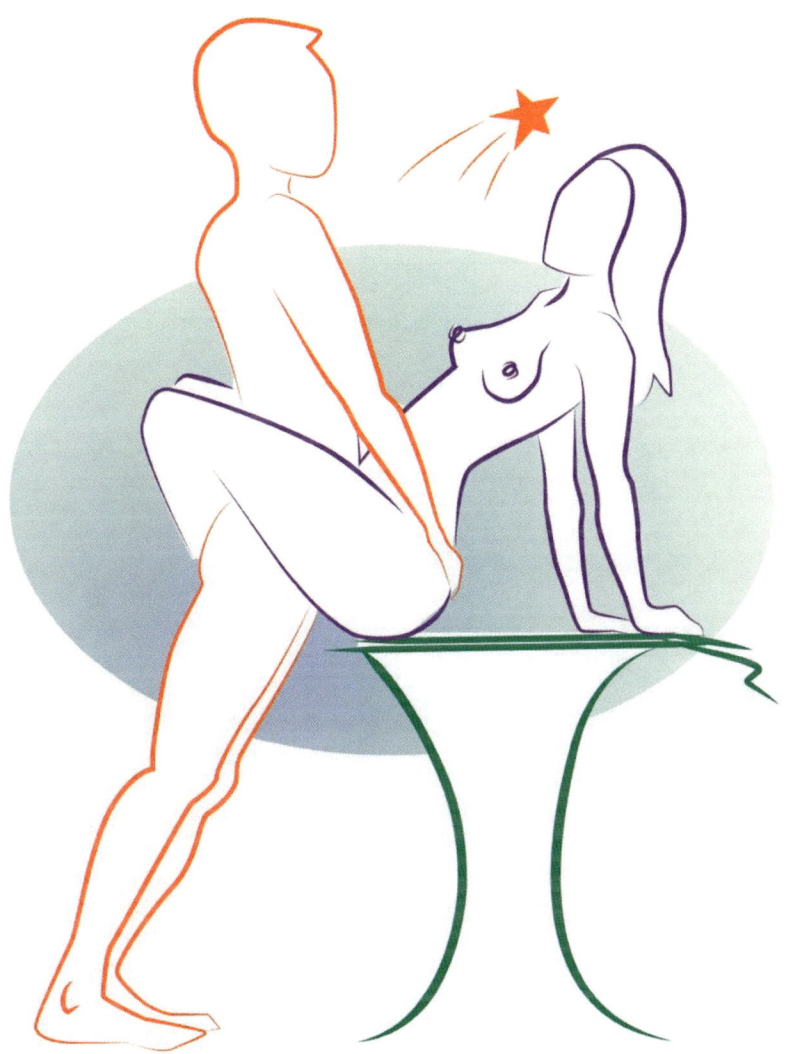

The *'Table Wrap'* is very easy even for the 50+ crowd.

Finding the right piece of furniture, the right height could be the only issue. But once that is solved what a great position for him to give her direct penetration.

As noted in the diagram, she climbs onto the sturdy high surface (we will say table). He moves to push into her as she wraps her legs firmly around his hips. She can squeeze him to let him know she wants him deeper in her or loosen so both can watch as he pulls himself out of her and pushes back into her. An orgasm in this position is pure delight for both.

'Lovers Embrace'

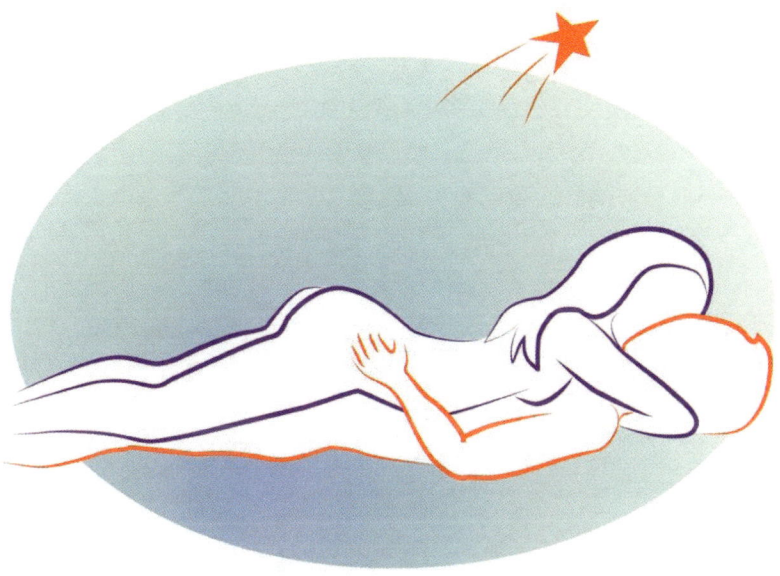

In the *'Lovers Embrace'* position the man lies on his back, the woman lies on top with her legs together. While he penetrates her she begins to rub up and down his body. The slide sex position is pretty easy to master and he'll be surprised at how much tighter she feels! This position is also great in the reverse with the man on top. He will come quickly in this position because of her tightness.

'Sideways Visit'

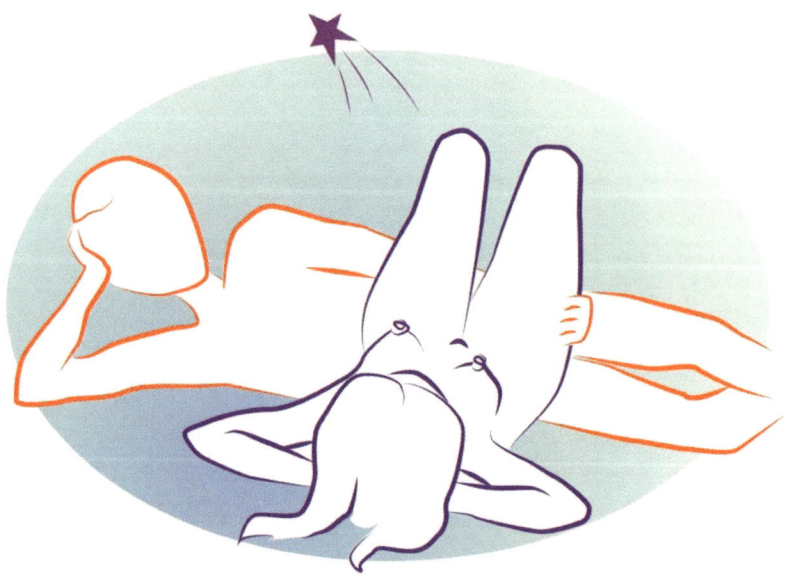

The *'Sideways Visit'* is a good resting position, ideal for getting your breath back during a long session. Her hands are free for caresses and she can enjoy the intimacy of gazing into her partners eyes. She lies back and he lies on his side at a right angle to her. She puts her knees over his hip to allow gentle penetration.

'Botty Brace'

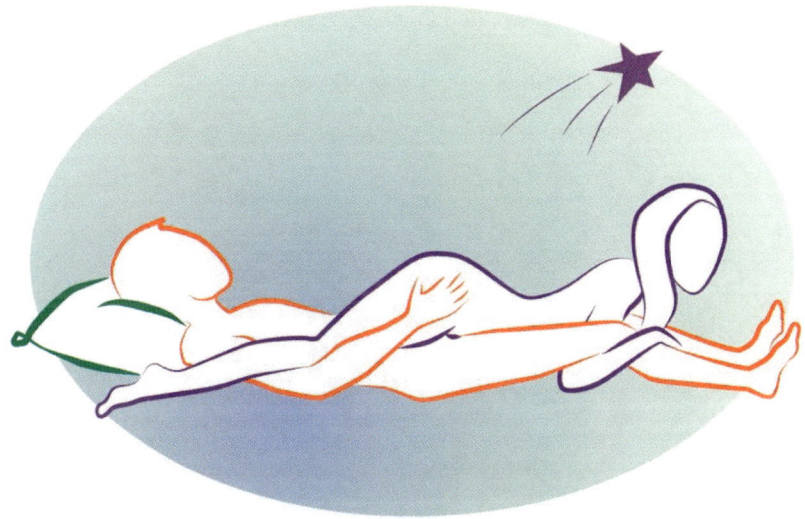

The *'Botty Brace'* with her Brown Eye provides him the delight of fondling her and rubbing her sphincter to her total enjoyment. He will need to lie face up with a pillow/cushion under his head. She moves to lie on top of him with her head at his feet and her legs extended on outside of each shoulder. He slides into her, as she wraps her arms around his calves to give her the leverage to push for deeper and deeper penetration into her as each gets into a rhythmic stroke. She may want to push with her toes to feel a more aggressive penetration into her.

'Tight Squeeze' of the Fondle

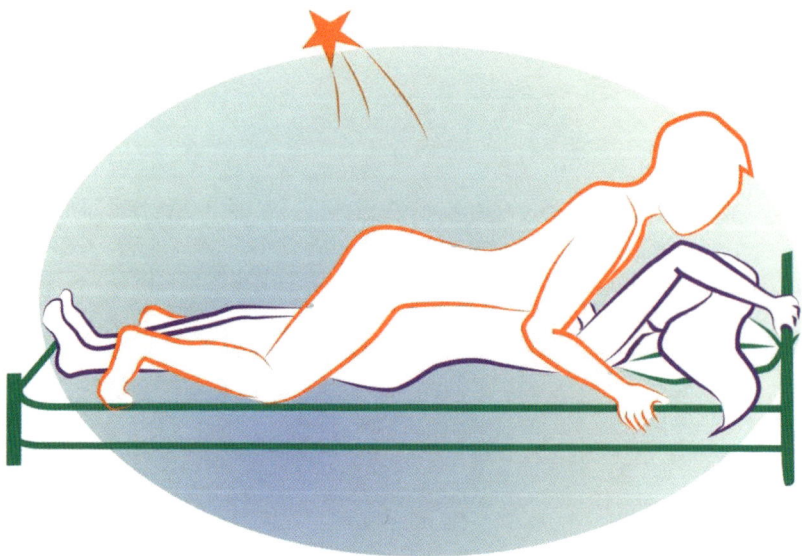

It is a very 'Tight Squeeze ' that will provide a mutual stimulation from the pressure of him pushing inside her against her clitoris area literally with his shaft rubbing against her magic spot.   Start by her lying on her back with legs stretched out as she is holding onto the bed post giving her leverage to push him inside of her.   She keeps her legs together and he will enter her then tighten his tights that are outside of her thighs squeezing to add a natural pressure, rubbing himself and her clit with each harmonist stroke of his thrusting shaft.

'Love Triangle'

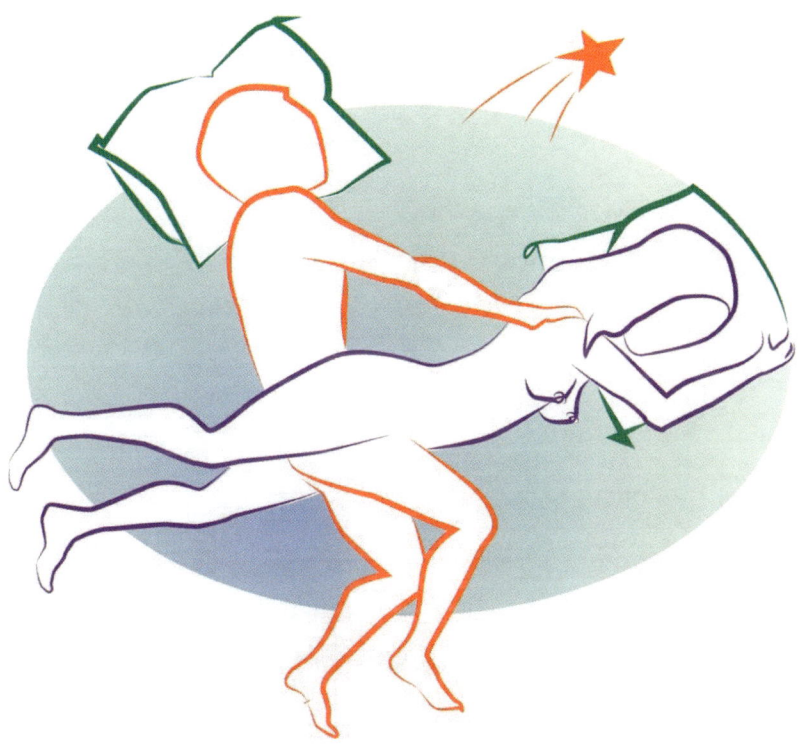

The 'Triangle' begins with both partners are on a bed or on the floor. She starts by lying on her side with her arms above her head. He lies on his side with his body perpendicular to hers. She raises her top leg so he can push himself in between her thighs. He holds her shoulders to give himself leverage for a gentle rocking motion. She can rub her clit as he strokes her breast or he can rub her clit as he moves in and out of her. Her orgasm will be quick and intense.

'Side Slider' and Massage

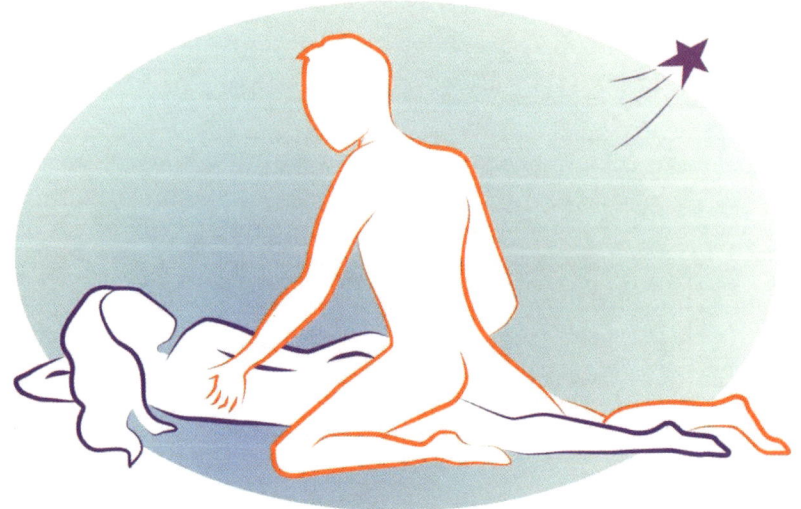

The *'Side Slider'* starts with her back to her partner as she lies down on her side. He kneels behind her facing towards her head. He slides the knee that's furthest from her head between her legs and then enters her. She moves her top leg and extends it slightly in front of her to give better balance and opening herself up to him. He also then has a better view. The side slide movement begins now as he holds on to her hips and thrusts into her. He can also gently massage her back and bottom.

'Secret Whispers' Expression of Desire

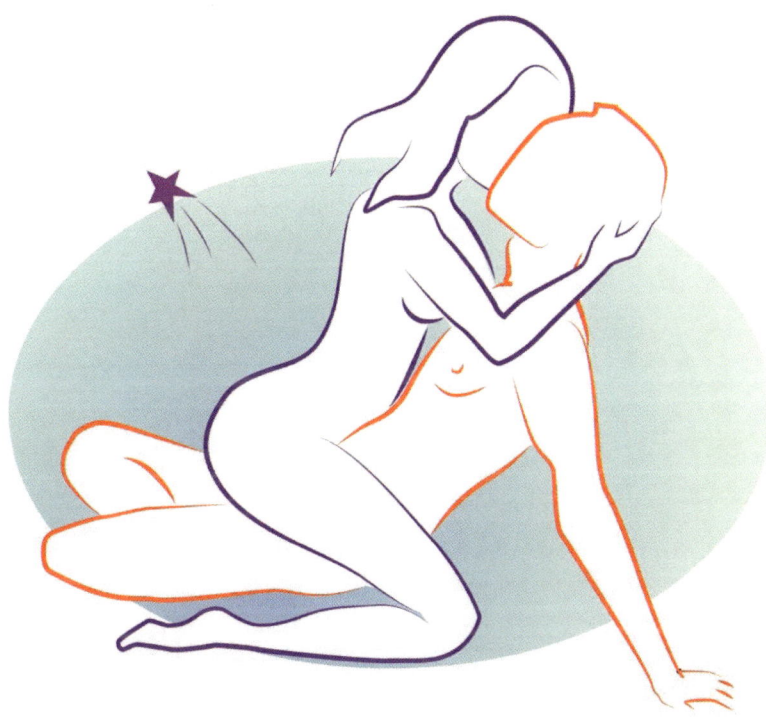

In 'Secret Whispers' he sits cross-legged leaning back supporting himself with both arms behind him. She kneels over his lap hugging him with her thighs and lowers herself down on to him. She can then determine the speed and depth of penetration. It may be easier to maintain the 'Secret Whispers' position for the man to lean against a wall or the edge of the bed and help her slide up and down, or just lean back and enjoy her lustful passion. She can whisper sweet secrets to her lover and gently nibble around his ears. This will drive the man for more......"tell me your secrets my love!"

'Brace & Push' of the Back Passage

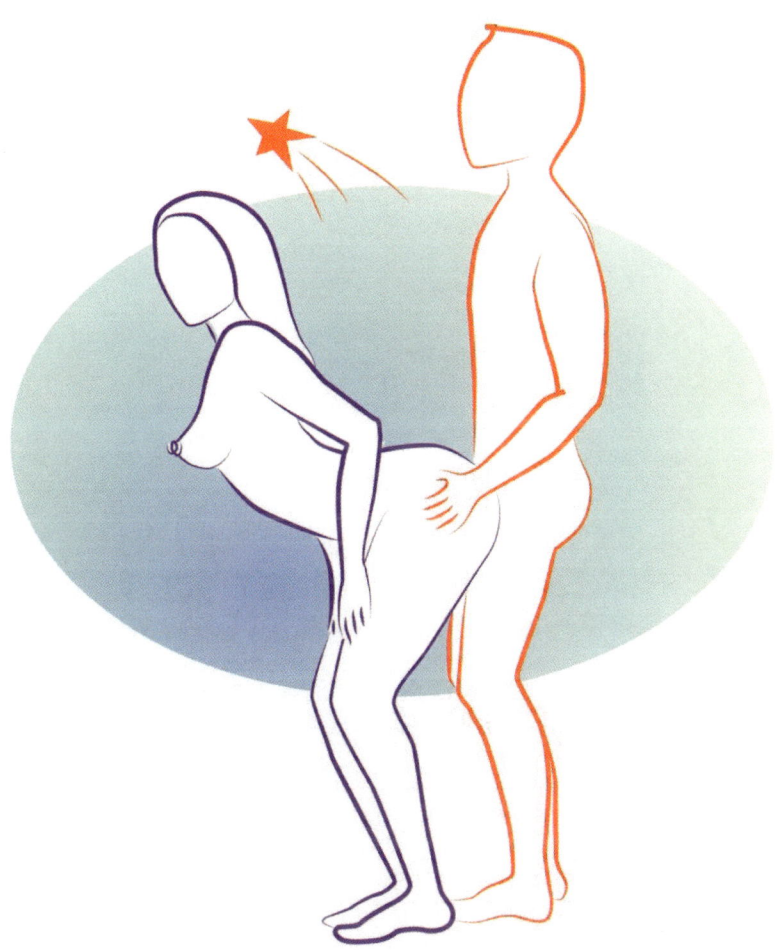

If she has a wall to lean against, the *'Brace and Push'* can give her more leverage to give that extra push as he moves in and out of her. The man stands up right and enters her from behind. He controls the thrusts as he holds onto her thighs. You can also perform the 'Brace and Push' sex position with him leaning against the wall. Ideal for anal penetration if that is one of your desires!

Kamasutra's 'Back Door'

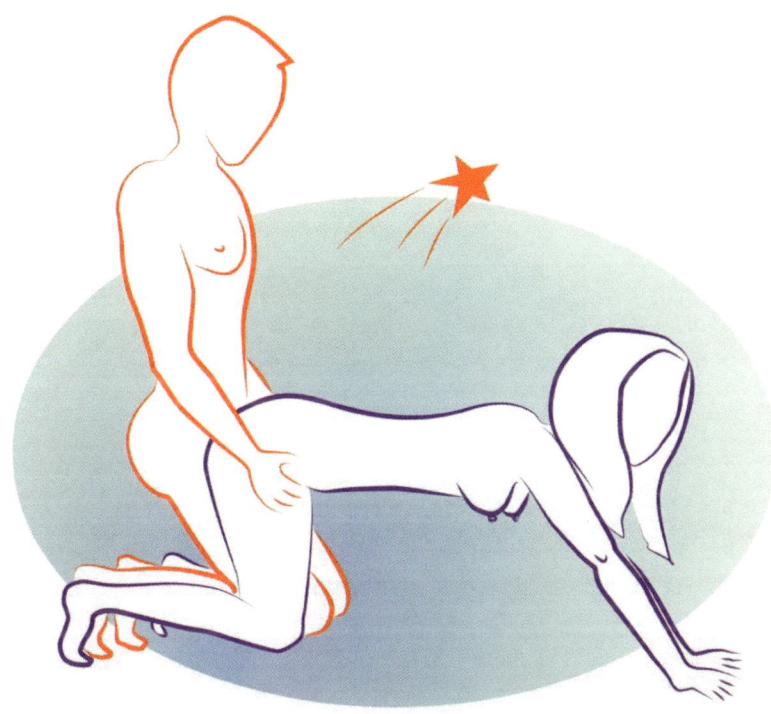

The 'Back Door', a type of doggy-style posture, is an absolute classic and like it or loathe it, it's one that's in every girl and guy's favorite repertoire.

We are sure the missionaries didn't like it, but that is probably because there is so much pleasure given by this sex position for both partners.

He kneels behind her as she positions herself on all fours. Holding her hips he inserts himself into her as she pushes back against him shifting her weight from her hands back towards her partner putting pressure against his shaft with each stroke. She can rock back and forth, push harder, increase the rhythm or verbalize her desires!

Cuddle 'Clit Stim'

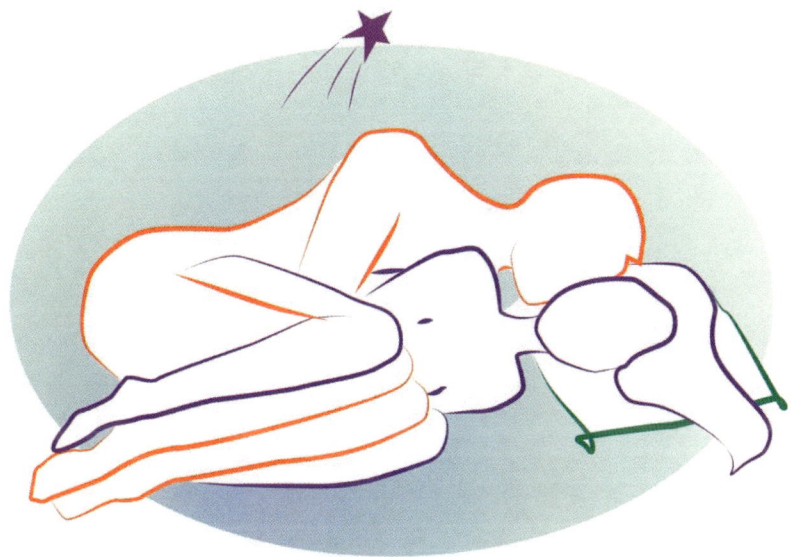

The *'Clit Stim'* is a variation on the simple 'Z' Embrace position. This close-up sex position is slightly more difficult to master. Lying on their sides he enters her from behind but this time she wraps her legs round the outside of his. They can both reach the clit for a good pre-penetration play or during penetration. He can also concentrate on her breasts while she pleases herself.

Warmth of 'The Wrap'

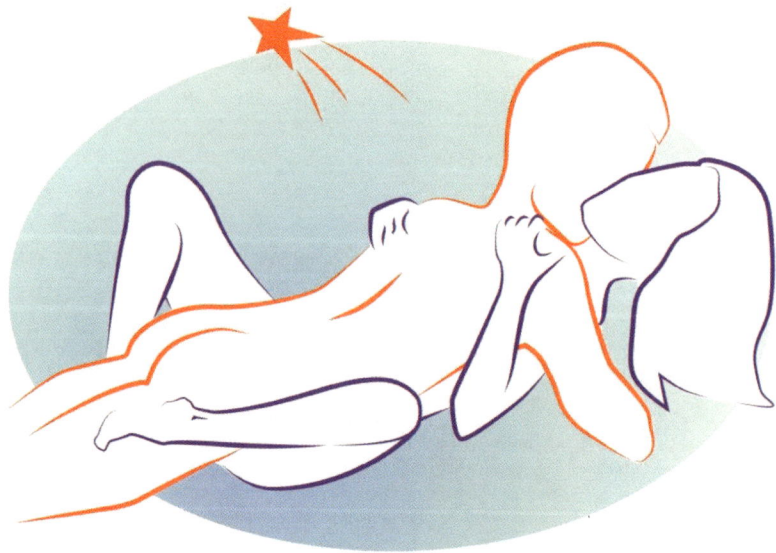

The *'Wrap'*, we all have experienced during our sexually active years. It begins with her lying on her back with her legs open exposing her pleasure spot. If she chooses, she can invite him to kiss her exposed lips to start her juices to flow and begin the ascent of her deep arousal. He moves to lie down, sliding between her legs entering her as she wraps her legs around his bottom pulling him deeper into her, literally locking him in her. Both partners can use their hands to stroke each other providing a very intimate lovemaking experience.

'Z Kamasutra Embrace'

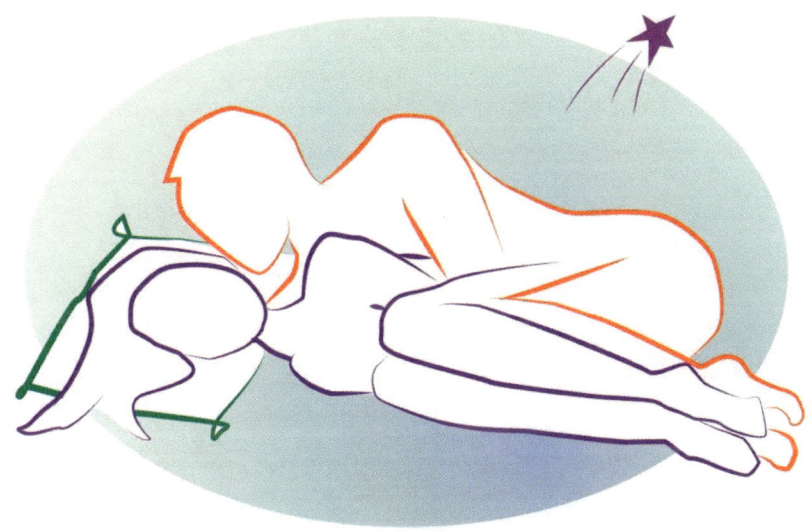

The *'Z-embrace'* is an easier variation of the 'Clit Stim'.
The woman curls up on her side, knees drawn up as he moves
his body to mirror her snuggling as close as he, skin to skin, as
he enters her from behind.   Penetration is fairly easy from his
position and the man can reach around to play her breasts or
clit.   She can also stimulate herself as well as request anal
penetration!   Very close, sensuous lovemaking.

'Reaching for Pleasure' inside the Kamasutra

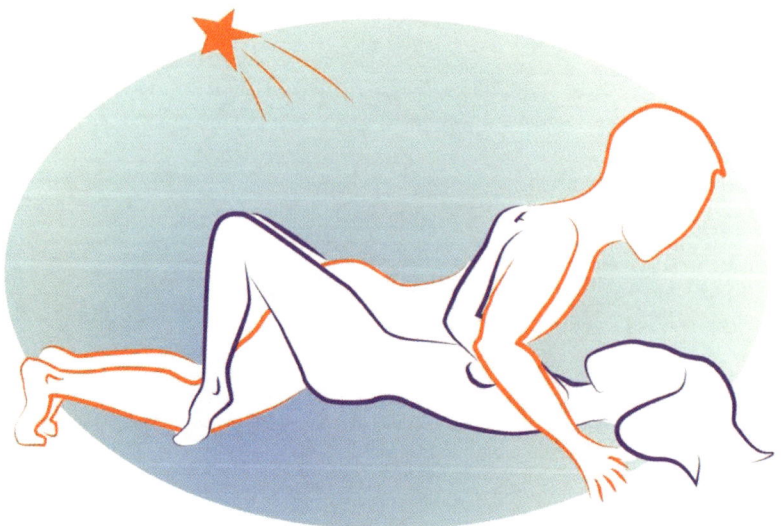

'Reaching for Pleasure', she is on her back and the man on top. He must balance himself on his knees and hands raising his hips so his stiffness becomes available to her as she lifts her hips pushing, receiving him inside her. He can push slightly to help with the penetration into her. She will naturally take control thrusting upwards experiencing more of him and pleasure for both with each stroke. He must maintain his position letting her control the stroking inside her with her hips thrusting movement.

Erotic 'Bamboo Split'

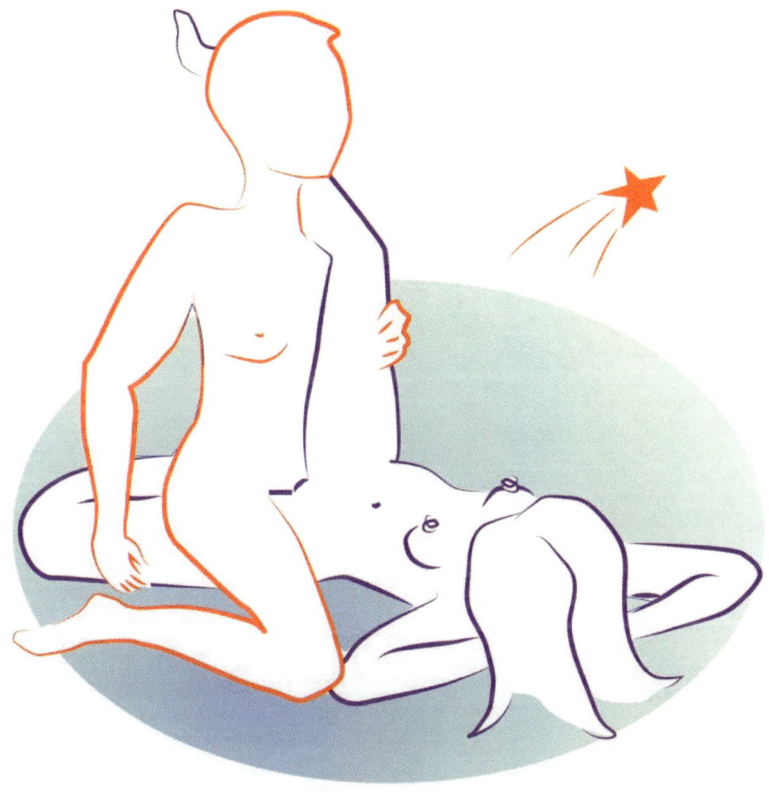

'Bamboo Split' is a classic Kamasutra position where the man is in control and she is free with her hands to stroke and stimulate her clitoris pleasuring herself while exciting him more as he pushes into her and pulls out to push again into her as she strokes herself. She lies on her back with a leg over his shoulder. He straddles her other thigh and enters her supporting himself with one hand against her thigh and bracing

himself on her raised leg. He can then move himself in and out of her and she can stroke her clit; a magnificent 'turn-on' for both!

'Lustful Lean'

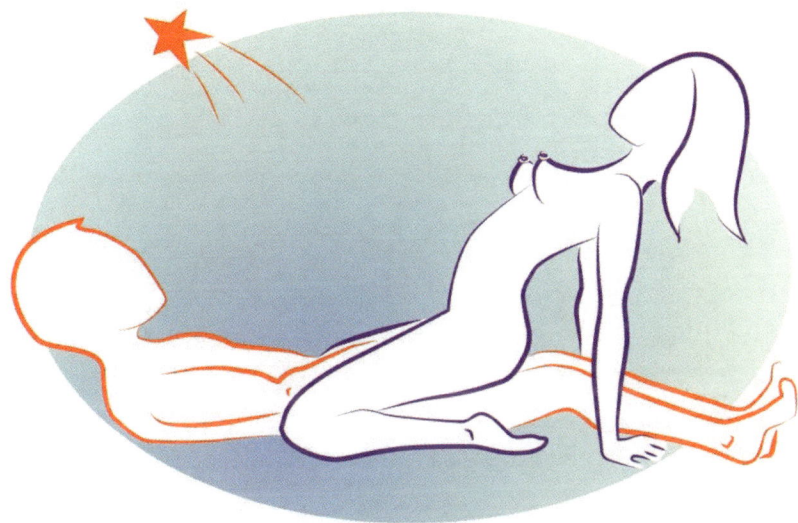

   'Lustful Lean' is another Kamasutra known to all followers of this art form.   He positions himself on his back with legs closed.   She pushes his rigid shaft inside of her as she sits down on him.   Once he's inside her as deep as possible, she leans back for support using her arms and hands.   She then creates a rhythm of movements to push into her more and from side to side as the man watches her actions and stimulates her clit.   The sway of her breasts and the stretching of her body in this position is very stimulating.

'Squatting Tigress'

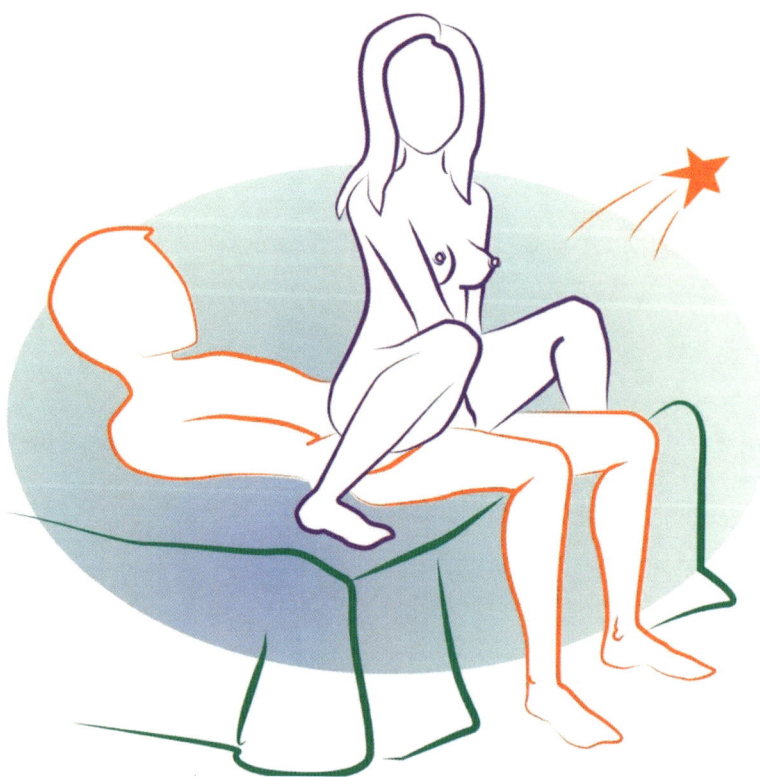

'Squatting Tigress' has always been a position synonymous with the art of Kamasutra; a position that requires the support of both parties. Highly erotic position for her especially when using a mirror to watch her movements. He lies on his back on the bed with his knees on the edge and feet on the floor. She squats on him, facing away sliding both feet under her in a squatting stance as he becomes secure in her. He places his hands under her bottom to help support her movements up and down on him, as she starts her movements by pulling up

exposing his shaft then moving down watching it disappear inside of her. She can balance herself with one hand, allowing her to fondle her clit or cuddle his balls with her other hand. She controls the depth and pace of penetration as he helps by lifting with each stroke on her bottom. This position is easier than it looks, as each partner strokes or touches the other.

'Hold and Cuddle' Tenderness

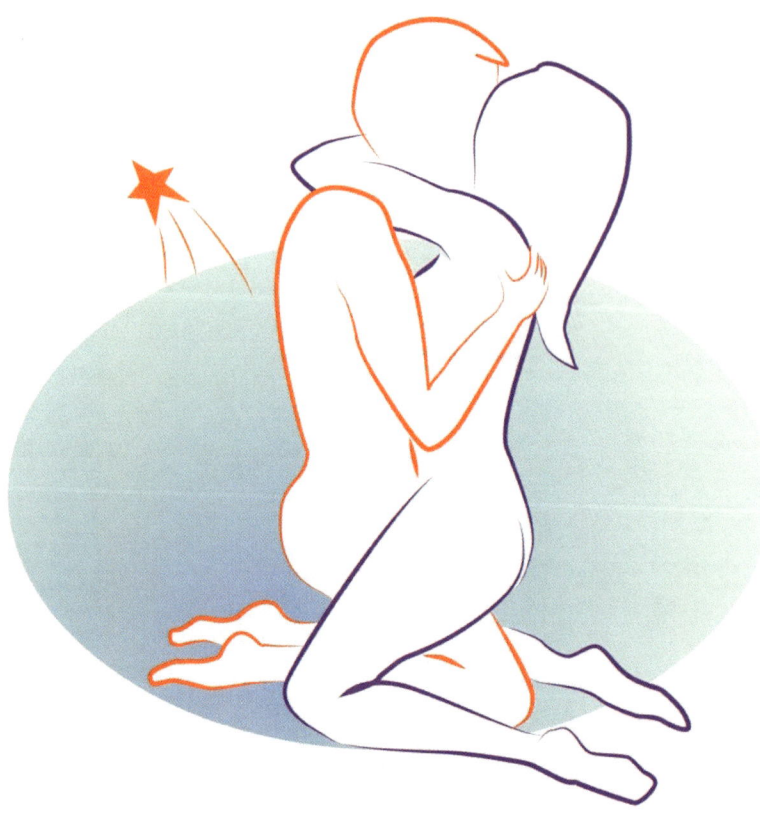

The woman and man kneel face to face in the *'Hold and Cuddle'* sex position. She straddles his thighs so he can enter her and as she wraps her arms around his neck. He embraces her using the motion of his knees, moving gently up and down penetrating her with each push. A very intense physical feel to this position.

'Baby Love'

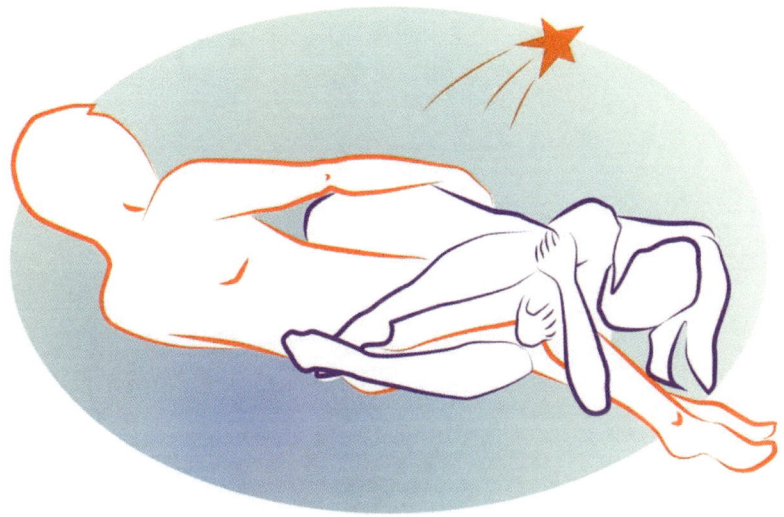

'Baby Love' is a much easier Kamasutra position than it looks. He starts by lying on his side. She curls up in a semi fetal position on her side in the opposite direction. Her head is at his feet. She pulls her knees up to her chest opening her thighs so she can sandwich his legs between them.

She holds on to his legs, pressing them against her breasts using her arms as he supports himself on his arm and elbow using his lose hand to guide himself into her. He can then start moving in and out of her, adding to her pleasure by using his free hand to stimulate her perineum and her anus. Very erotic, very lustful!

Classic 'Missionary' Pleasure

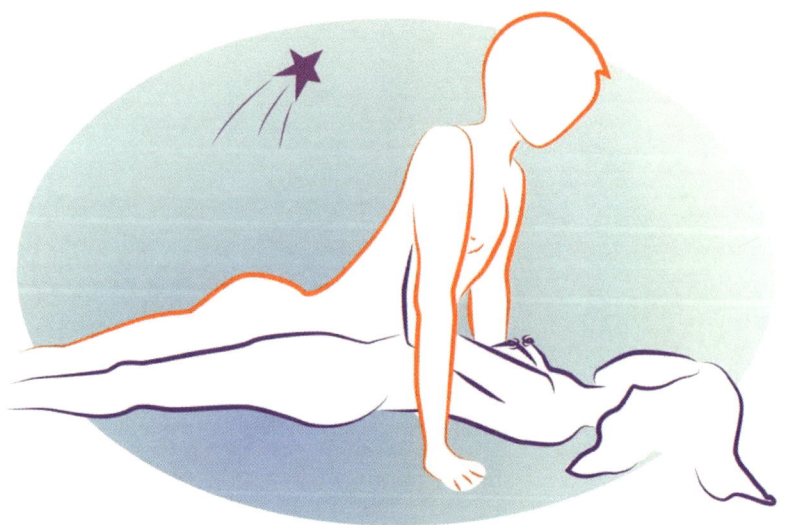

'Missionary' position is where we all started with the classic Kamasutra. I wonder if the missionaries read this in their Kamasutra handbook and decided to teach the flock that this is the most 'civilized' position for intercourse. Who knows, but it is fun to speculate. She is on her back with her legs slightly apart. He is on top between her thighs supporting himself on his arms so he can watch her. She can use her arms to pull him into her controlling the rhythm and depth of the stroke she likes. He easily slides in and out of her as she lies back and enjoys each stroke.

'Open Pleasure'

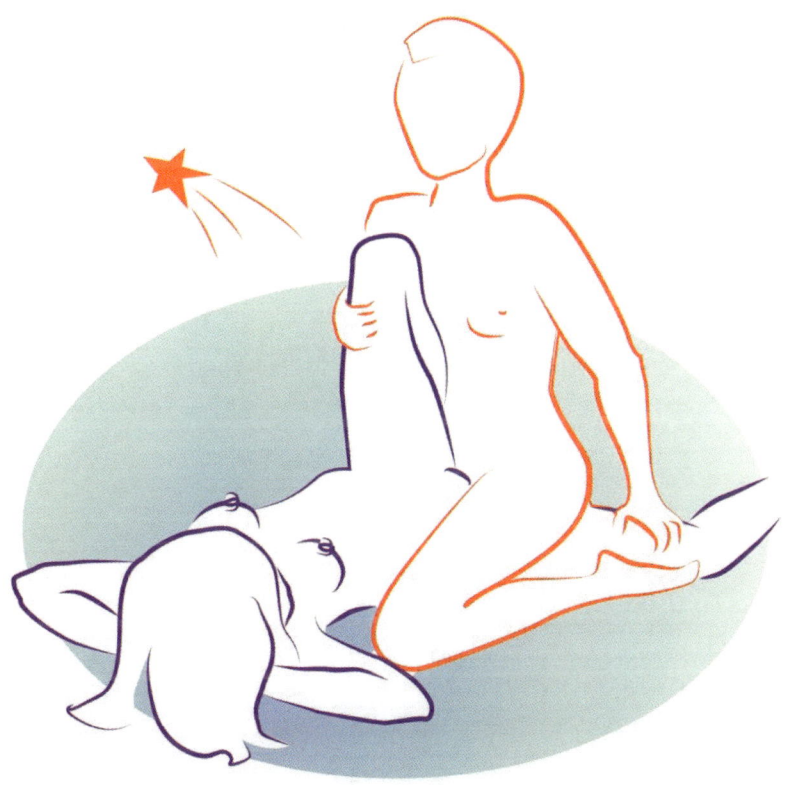

'Open Pleasure' is a restful position for her. Once inside
her he can push her bent leg to open her up for deeper
penetrating pleasure while she reclines holding her head up to
see when each stroke is moving into her. She starts by lying
on her back with a leg extended, the other bent up making sure
she has spread her thighs so he will have no problem entering
her. He will sits down on her thigh of the extended leg and
slips her bent leg under his arm. To begin with, he uses his

hand to brace himself as he guides himself between her thighs into her.   He then braces himself with that hand placing it behind him to support himself thus having complete control as he establishes the rhythm of his movement in and out of her.

'Cushioned Table'

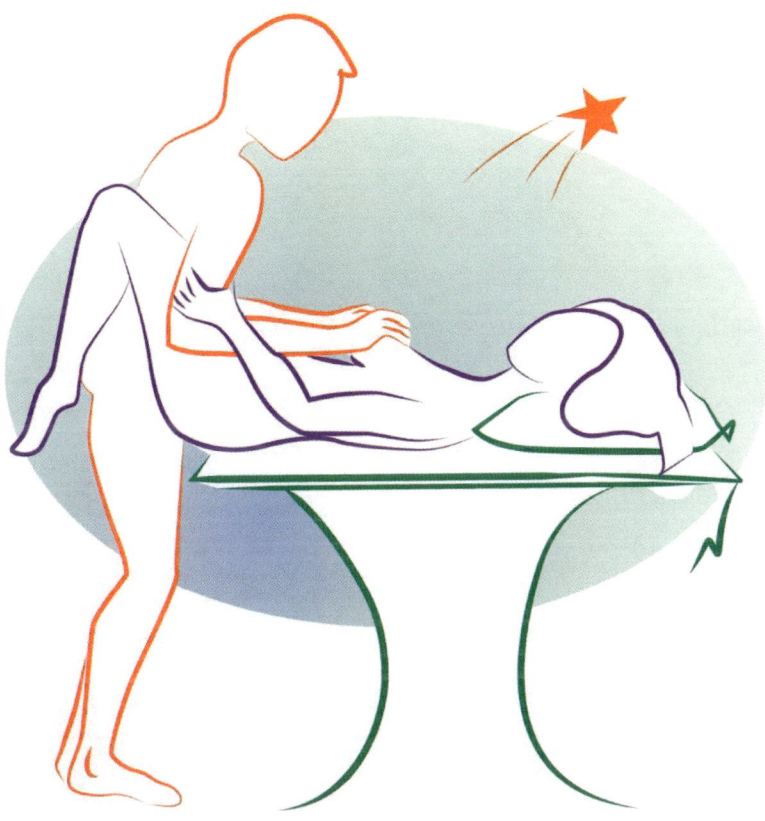

She lies on her back, with her bottom at the edge of the bed or table for the *Cushioned Table* sex position. Her partner enters her while caressing her breasts or clitoris. A good position also working well without thrusting: if the woman grips hold of the man by crossing her ankles behind his back and he presses himself against her, the pressure will mount; giving both partners intense pleasure, each generates an in and out thrusting motion that feels all natural. Also a very stimulating position for her to exercise her vaginal muscles as he is deep in her

'G Spot Massage'

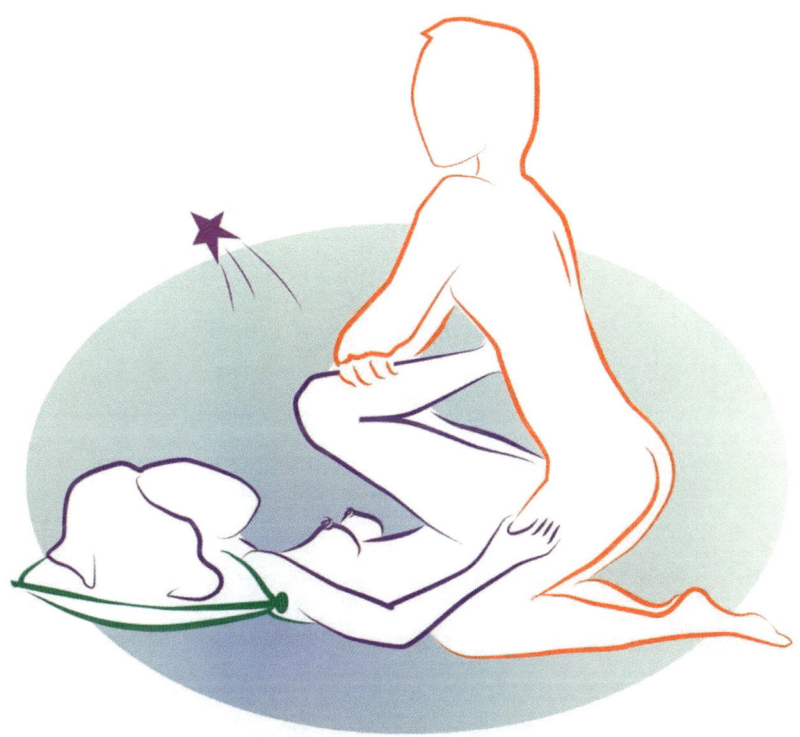

'G-Spot Massage' is a great Kamasutra position for him to use his penis to massage her G-spot. She starts by lying on her back pulling her knees to her chest. He kneels facing her placing her feet on his chest. He starts to penetrate her as he leans forward placing his forearms on her knees as she grips each of his thighs. She can now pull him closer making his penetration deeper into her. The G-spot massage starts with him adding pressure to the G-spot by pressing her knees down with his arms. The more pressure the more action for the G-

spot. He can look into her eyes watching her come to a point of ecstasy as he applies more and more pressure on her knees. Very pleasing for both.

'Rock-a-Bye-Baby'

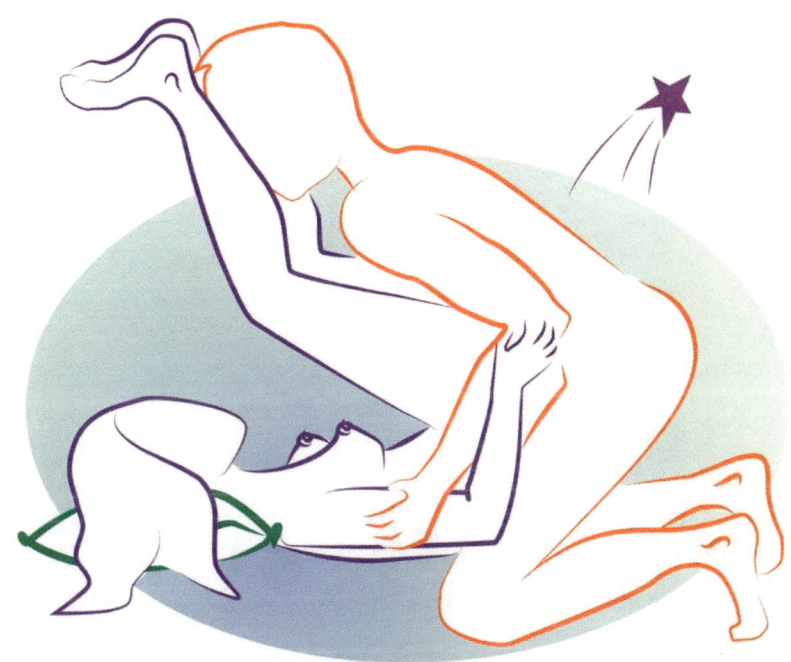

'Rock-a-Bye Baby' is a romantic name for a posture that allows him to fully penetrate her with all the depth of his manhood. She lies on her back and pulls her legs back over her head like she is going to do a backward somersault. He kneels down against her elevated hips and open thighs, pressing against her to help her to keep her legs back and her hips up. He now places himself between her lips and penetrates deep into her rocking back and forth. This position is ideal for anal penetration, if this is one of your pleasures.

Wondrous 'Sensual Spread'

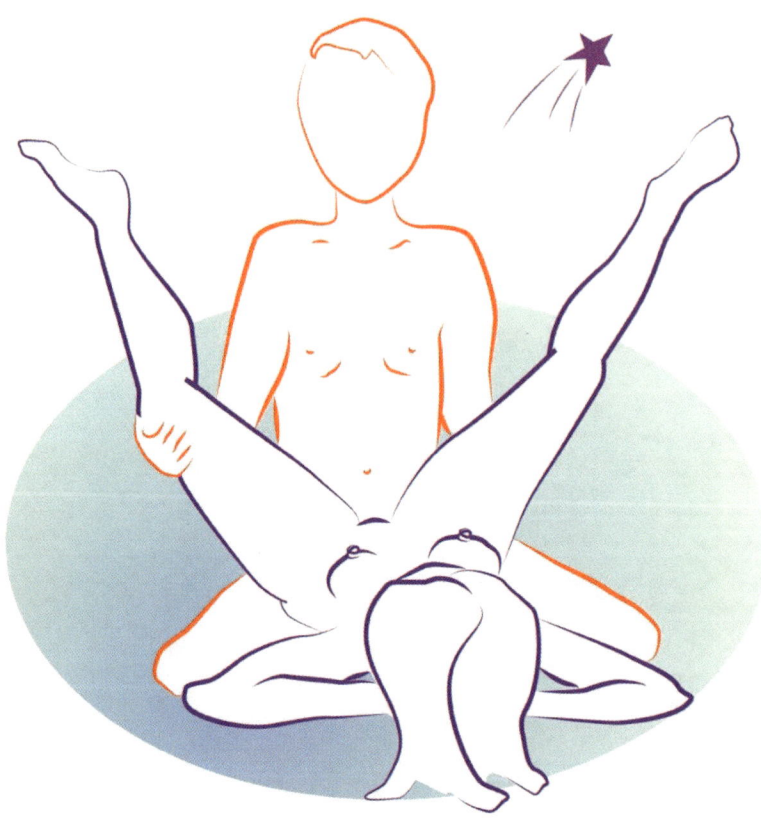

'Sensual Spread' another great Kamasutra position for him to watch his strokes into and out of her as she lays back and pleasures the action.   He spreads his legs sitting on his knees in front of her.   She lies on her back, usually with her head resting on a pillow.   Her legs are in the air and spread wide apart with him holding each leg as a balance for him and to ensure she can hold herself in that inviting position.   This will

enable her to relax a bit with him holding her legs up and apart. She is very exposed and open as he penetrates her; varying both the speed and depth of his strokes. She can relax as she enjoys his strokes. He in turn has a wonderful view of his actions in her. Real turn on!

'Stretch Hold and Bang' Stimulator

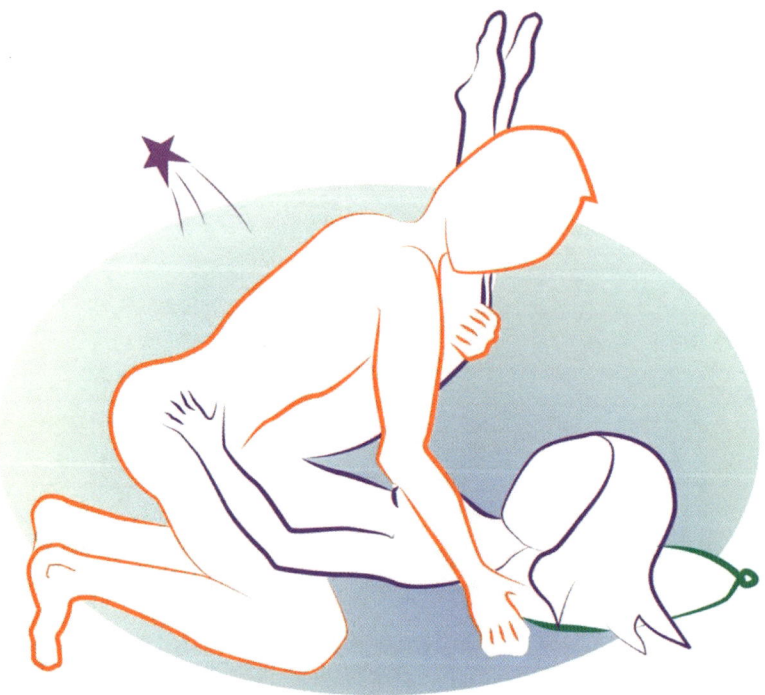

The *'Stretch, Hold and Bang'* requires her to lay back with a pillow under her head, her legs in the air as straight and high as possible. He kneels in front of her gripping both of her legs putting them over one of his shoulders. He leans forward, and enters her slightly off center. He can place his hand on the bed or floor for support. This is a rough and ready position, both need to be relaxed and the man thrust hard with his hips deep into her. Quite a spectacular position.

'Pleasure Stretch'

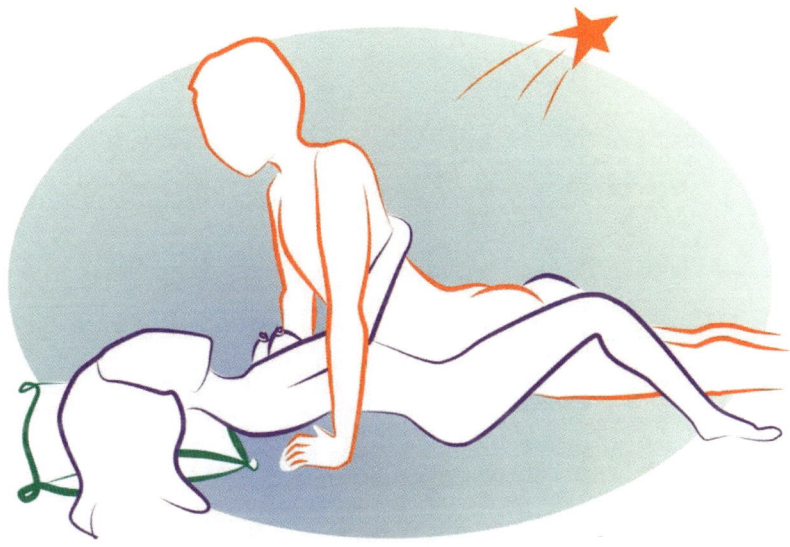

'Pleasure Stretch' is a wonderful position letting him have full access to her.   .She starts by lying on her back with legs open and a pillow under her head to view her partner, and under her bottom pushing her hips up exposing her to make his penetration easier and deeper into her.   He moves over her, supporting himself with his arms.   She then places her hands on his him, his back and bottom supporting his thrusts into her. She can arch more to meet his strokes while looking into his eyes showing the pleasure he is giving her as she moves with him to lengthen each stroke.

'Deep Rhythm' Song

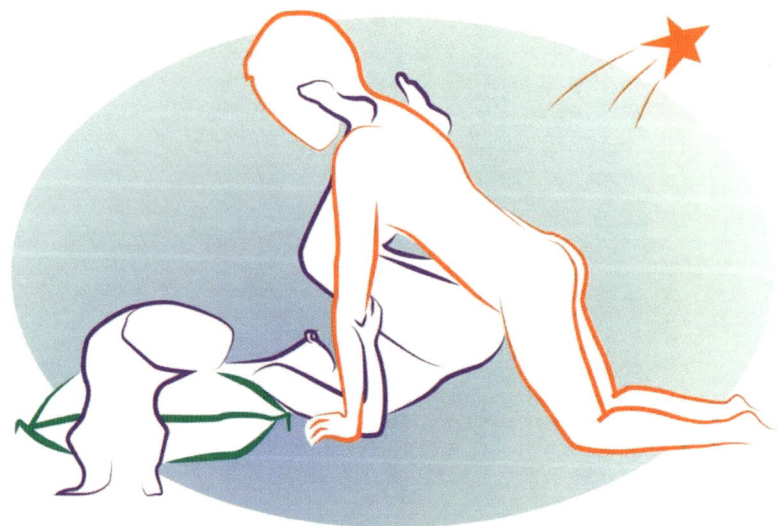

'Deep Rhythm' is a position for those who like very deep penetration. She will love this if she favors very deep insertion into her but what lover doesn't like deep penetration? Lying flat she pulls her knees into her chest touching her breasts. She then places her feet over her partner's shoulders that is kneeling in front of her. He enters her, putting his weight on his hands placed on either side of her shoulders. She is totally exposed and will naturally widen her thighs as she becomes more moist as the pace quickens. She will feel more stimulation when he reaches ejaculation and deepens each thrust as he ejaculates; very seductive and very erotic.

Also excellent position for anal penetration if that is in your repertoire.

'Side Snuggle' Love

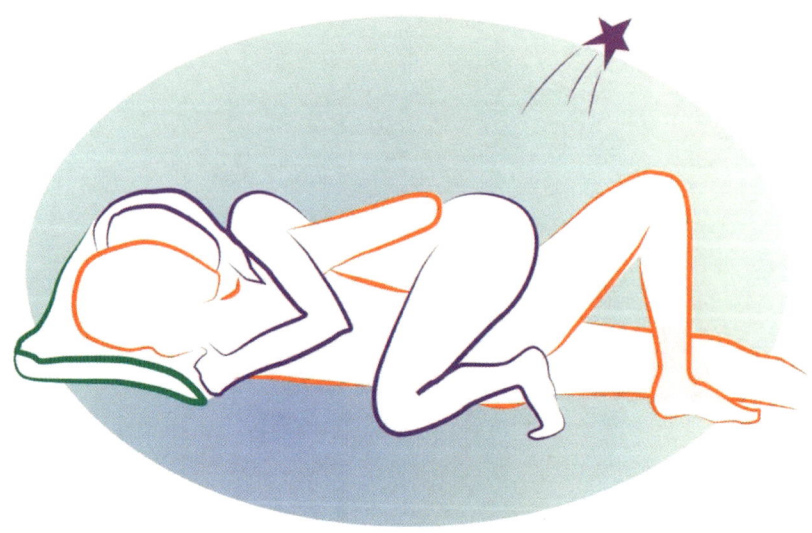

    'Side Snuggle' sex position can result from a cuddling embrace, a quiet moment of touching to him penetrating her, both feeling the closeness and joy of each other. When on the brink of the Big Orgasm, slow it down pushing deeper then again slides in and out totally feeling each other's tightness as you both approach an orgasm. Both roll onto their sides, face-to-face (if possible, he stays inside her the entire time), then put the passion on a low simmer with legs intertwined and chests pressed against one another. Slowly build back up to an even more incredible climax.

'Stairway to a Heavenly Orgasm

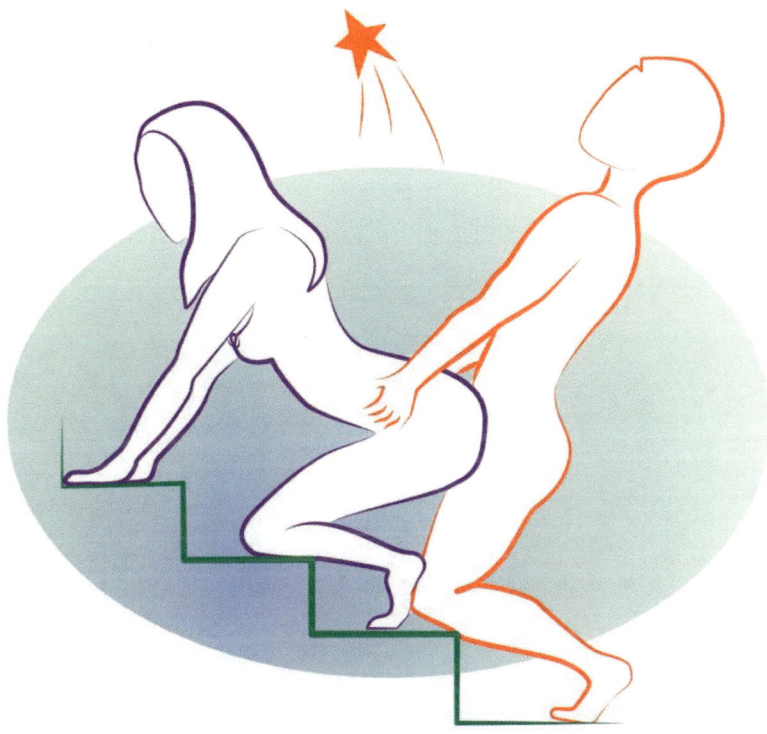

You need stairs with soft carpeting for the *'Stairway to Heaven'* sex position. She kneels in front of her partner on the staircase (choose the lower stairs!). While she reaches up to hold on to each side of the banister for support (or to the stairs themselves), he holds her hips and penetrates her from behind. A great position for anal sex if that is part of your repertoire.

'Pushing Embrace'

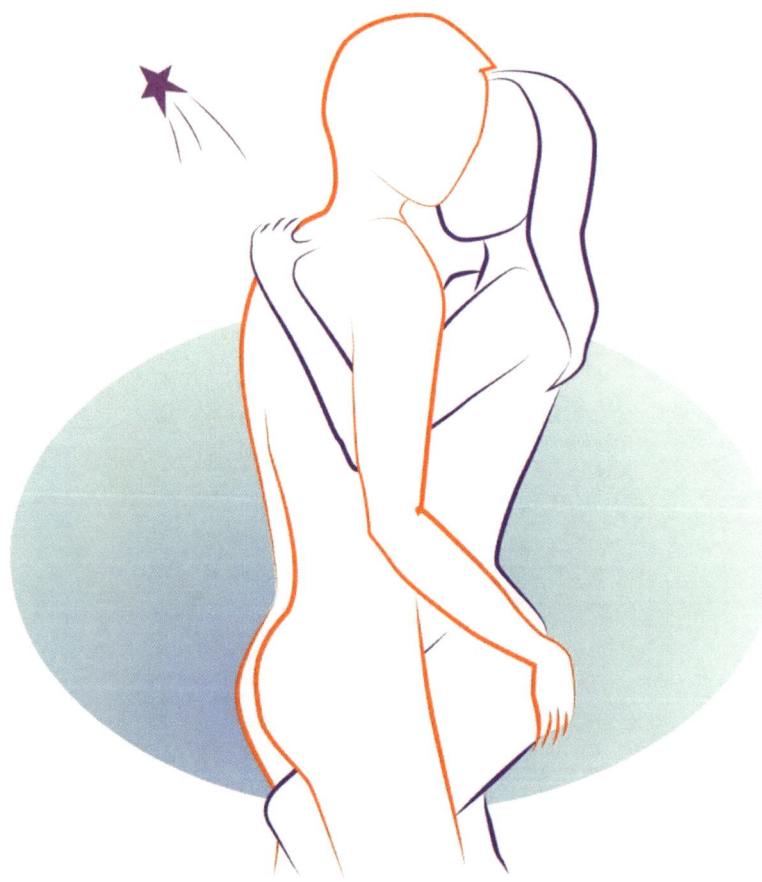

The *'Pushing Embrace'* sex position is a great position for impromptu sex especially a surprise greeting of your partner anytime, anywhere. Standing face to face, the man stimulates his partner's genitals with his penis and then penetrates her. This is easier if the woman is wearing heels or a similar height to her partner. If not, a table or work surface at the required height will do the trick! Very sensual stroking of each other will provide total skin stimulation. A great position to start, but the excitement can take you anywhere, against the wall, to the floor..., but all is good!

'Rocker'

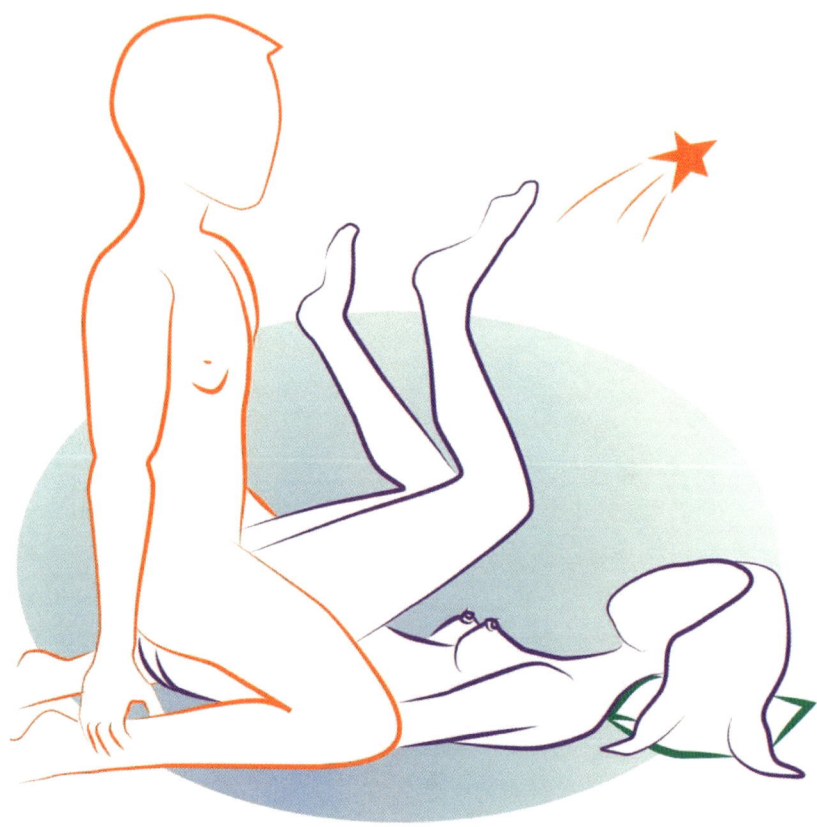

The 'Rocker' position gives deep penetration. Keeping legs up can be a challenge and need help as the movements become intense. The woman lies on her back with her head on a pillow and her pelvis raised by another pillow on the edge of the bed. She rocks back and draws her knees into her chest so her partner, kneeling in front of her, can enter her pushing gently into her wetness. As his pace quickens he can use his hands to stroke the backs of her thighs and help her hold her legs and hips up for deeper penetration.

'Stand & Deliver' Embrace

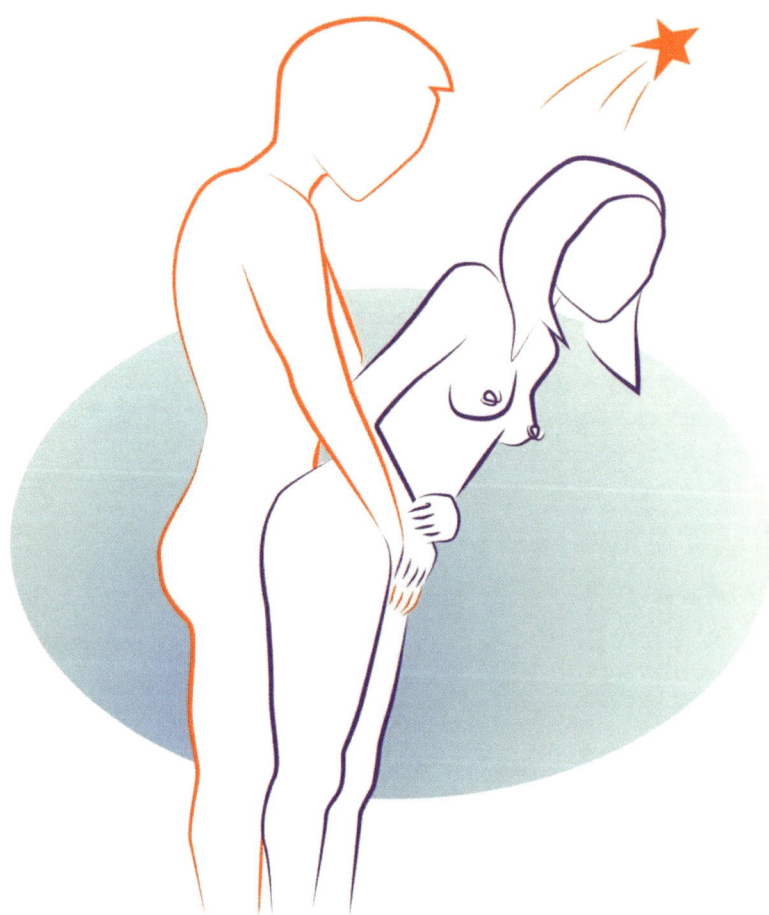

For the 'Stand & Deliver' both partners are standing, she is in front with her back to her partner, arms intertwined to maintain balance. He enters her from behind while she arches her back. She can also lean forwards onto a wall or table to allow deeper penetration and make things a little easier. Both can stimulate her clit making for a full blown standing orgasm.

'Sneakie'

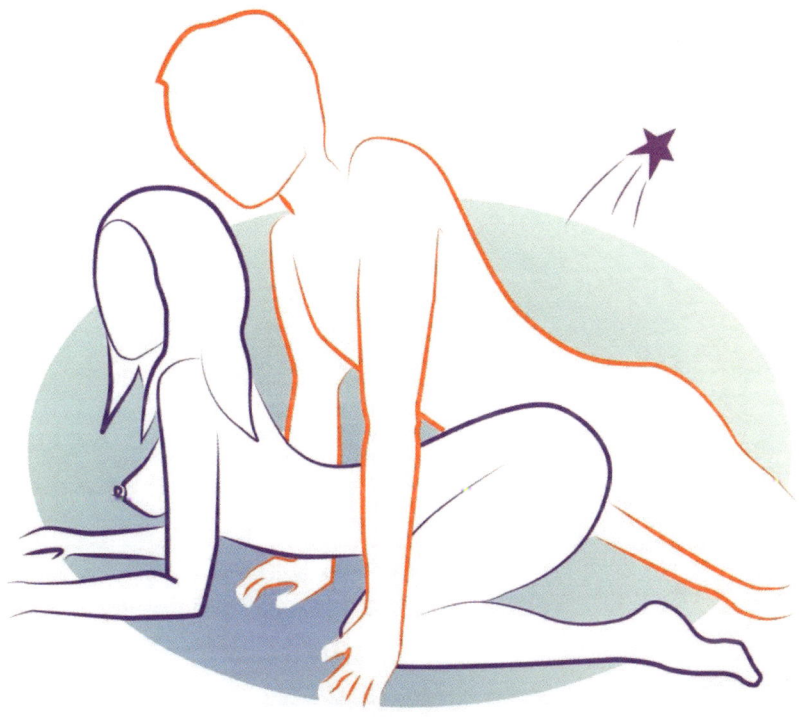

'Sneakie' has him sneaking up behind her as she is lying totally naked on her tummy in bed. She senses him approaching her and raises herself up placing her weight on her forearms comes to her knees but making sure she has exposed herself for him to enter her. She then bends one leg out to the side putting her now totally wet spot in full view for him as an invitation to continue his crawl toward her with his manhood ready to move into her. She keeps her other leg outstretched still on her knee. He crawls on top of her entering her from

behind keeping his weight on his arms as he moves deeper into her.

He adds pressure by relaxing his weight a bit as their skin melts together more with each thrust into her. As the rhythm and depth of strokes increase both will want this to last forever, it is that good.

Stimulation of the 'Rising'

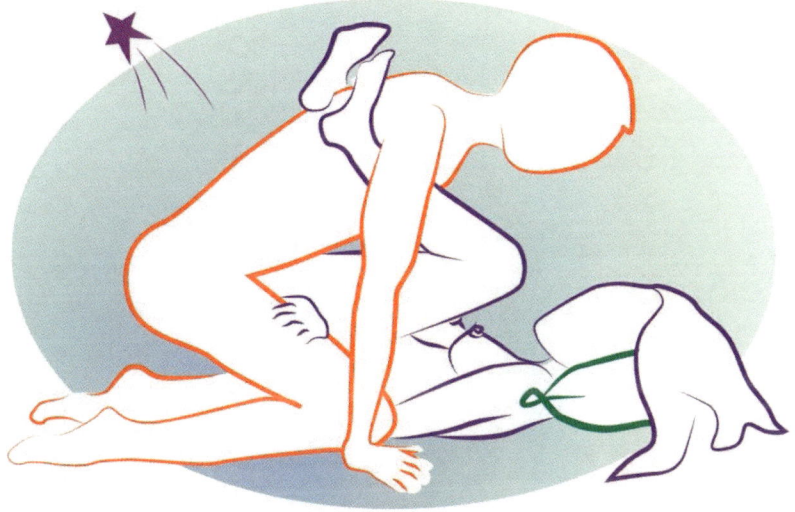

In the 'Rising' position she lies on her back with her knees bent up to her chest.   Her man then kneels down facing her and enters her.   She pulls him towards her by clasping her hands behind his bum and rests her legs by his armpits.   If the man is quite well endowed, this position will make it easier to 'accommodate' him.   The cushion gives her full view of their stroking together.

'Thigh Master' Workout

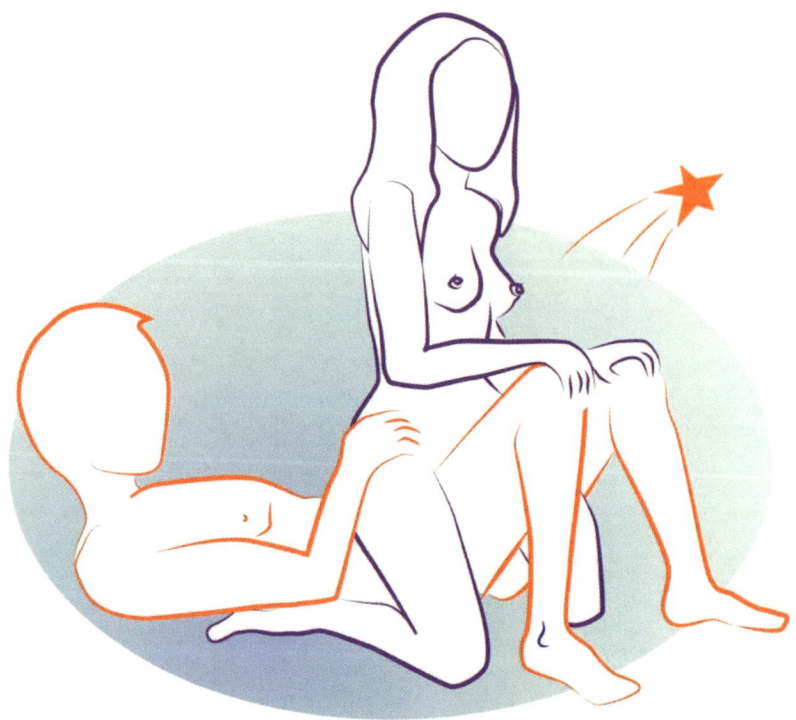

The 'Thigh Master' begins with him lying on his back with his legs bent up and apart. She straddles one of his thighs with her back to him. She holds on to his knee and lowers herself onto him. Her stomach is almost touching his bent knee; she can use it for support and leverage as she rocks back and forth and pushes up, then lowers herself down on him. She is in control.

'Flex&Stretch', Son of Kamasutra

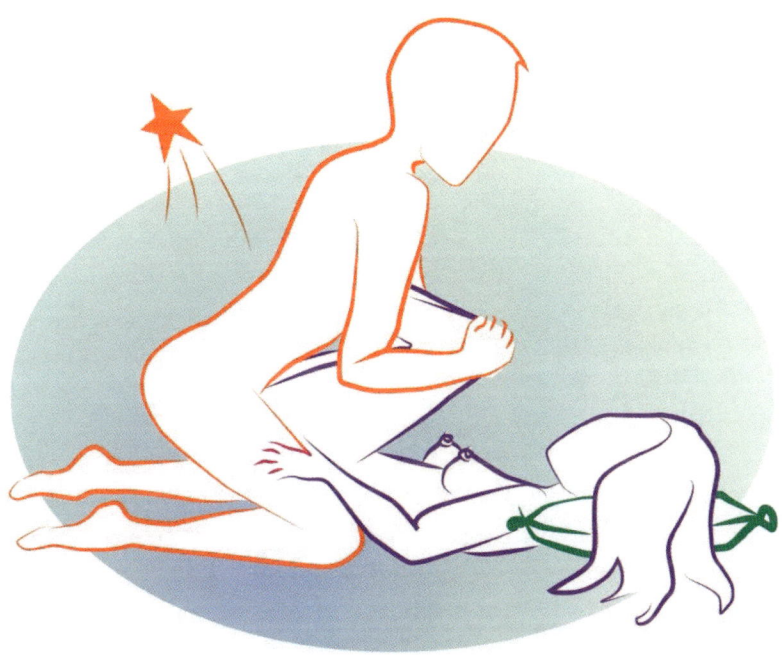

The 'Flex&Stretch' Kamasutra posture.   She is lying on her back with a cushion under her head pulling her knees up to her chest fully exposing herself to him.   The man kneels facing her moving to penetrates her.   She then places her feet against his chest.   He controls the thrusting, while his partner has her hands free to wander all over his body.   Penetration is very deep with the 'Flex & Stretch' position.

'Stirrup Ride' Bang

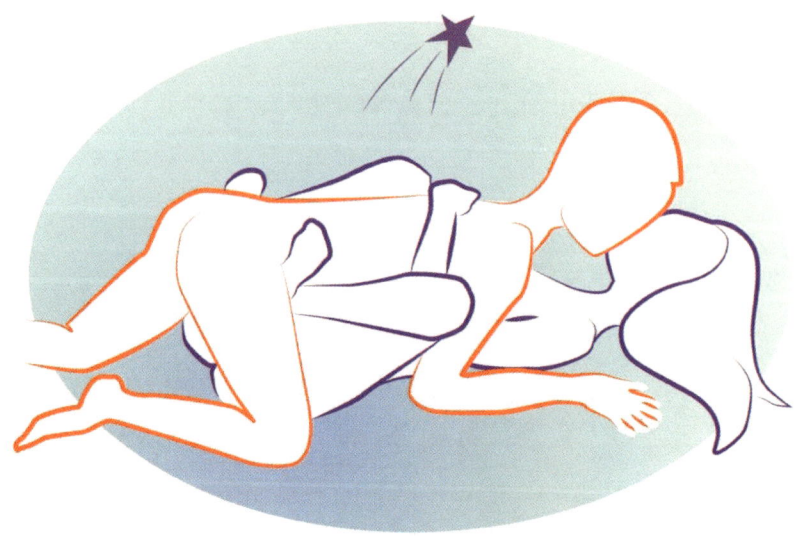

For the *'Stirrup Ride'* sex position, a little yoga practice could help especially for the woman to allow her hips to bend and flex.   She lies on her back, legs crossed just like the "lotus" position in yoga (the opposite foot on top of the opposite knee).   It may be advantageous to place a pillow or cushion under the small of her back.   He places himself between her legs lying gently on her now crossed legs, penetrating her exposed wetness, gently at first or very forceful, whatever her pleasure dictates.   Her total exposure will allow him to give her full strokes at a pace encouraged by both.   He will need to place most of his weight on his out stretched hands as he pushes into her and pulls out to push in again. Very sexy for him to see her totally exposed to his penetration. Forceful orgasms always follow, so beware!

'Cushion Pump'

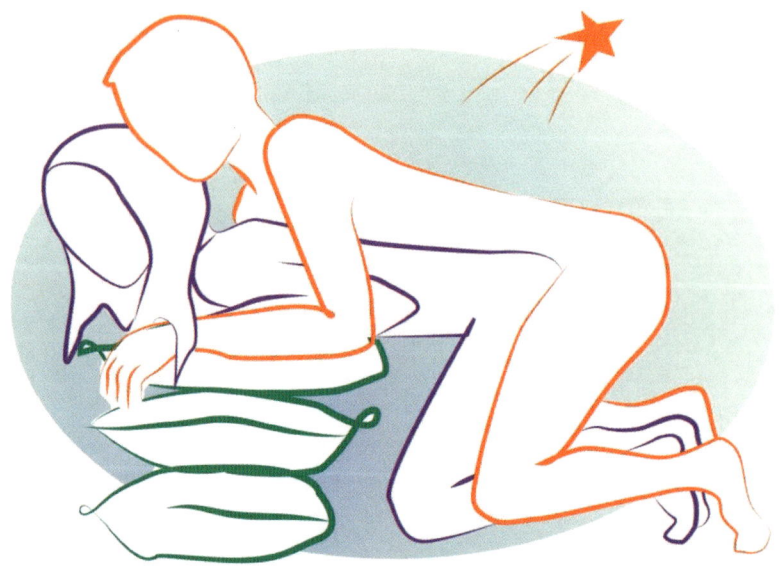

For the *'Cushion Pump'*, first of all construct your "mountain" out of a pile of pillows. The woman kneels in front of the pillows and leans forward over it. He kneels behind her, legs on the outside of hers; he leans down over her and penetrates her from behind. Make sure you use fairly firm pillows for this sex position as the going may get very bouncy. Very deep penetration and extremely comfortable for the woman!

'Her Chance' Erotica

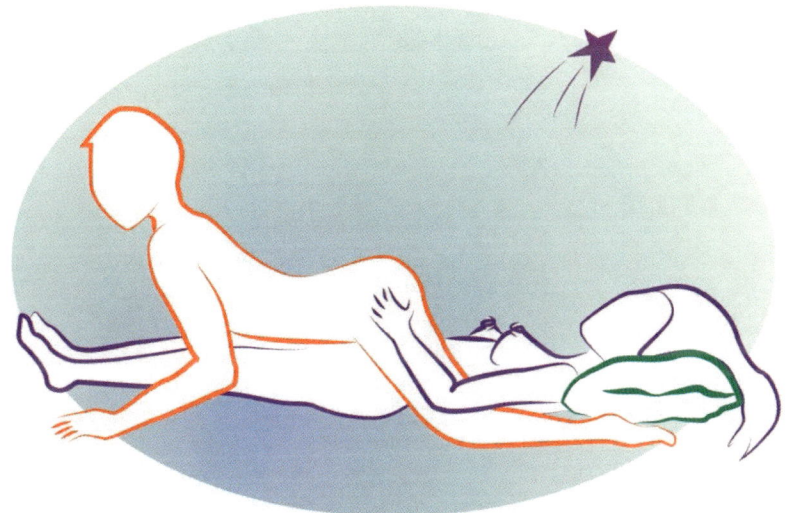

The 'Her Chance' is unusual. The Propeller sex position requires the woman to lie on her back - legs outstretched and together. The man lies on top of her but back-to-front so he's facing her feet. Once he's got himself inside he can make circular motions with his hips. This takes some practice to get right... we're not sure it's worth the effort unless she gets turned on by his ass and anus. It gives her a chance to anally stimulate him should he desire this!

'Deep Thrust' Pleasure

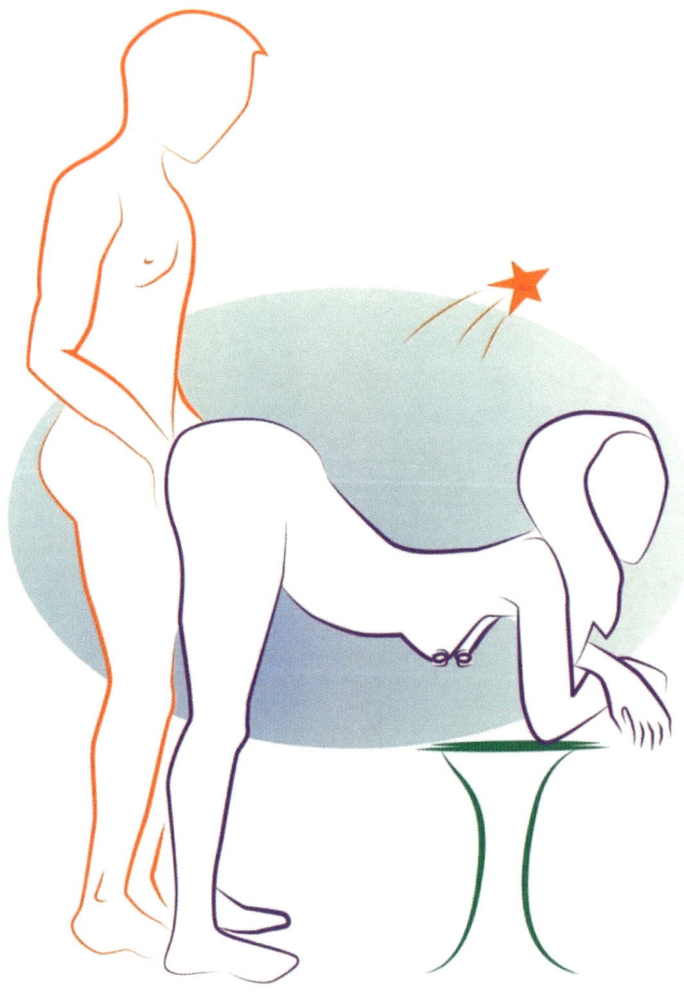

The woman stands with her back to her partner in the *'Deep Thrust'* sex position. She bends her knees and rests them on the edge of a chair or stool and crosses her arms on the back of the chair or on the stool to support herself. He enters her from behind and controls the movement, caressing her clitoris and breasts with his hands.   Penetration will be deep, stimulating the front walls of the vagina and G spot.   This is also a great position for anal sex or just anal finger stimulation.

'Side-Show'

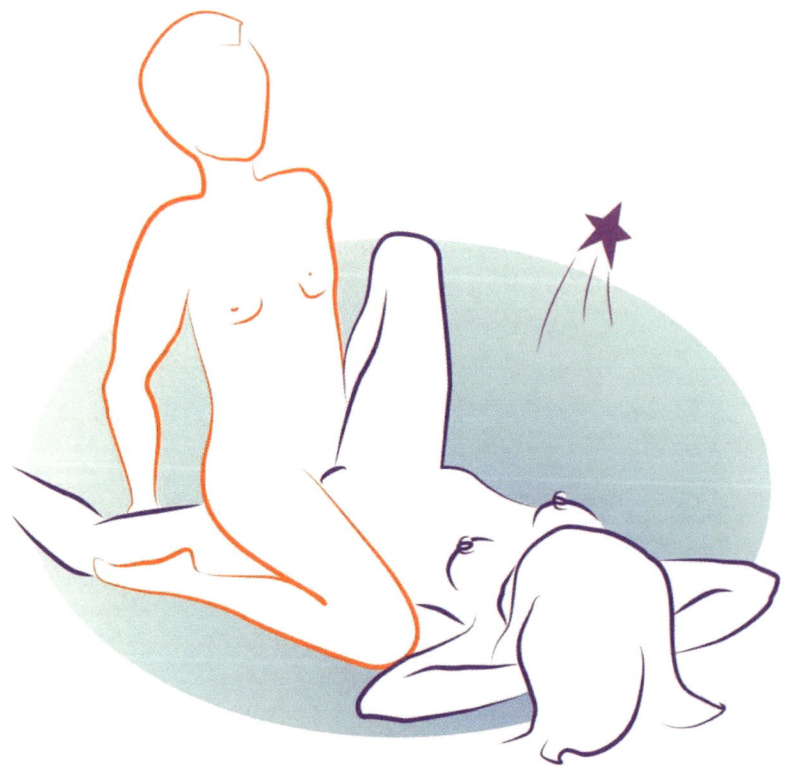

In the *'Side Show'* position she lies on her back, one leg bent up with the other leg lying flatly on the ground. He sits down between her legs and pushes a leg under her behind lifting and supporting her hip. Leaning back he braces himself with his hands behind his back. She has her hands free to play. She could also prop her head up to watch the action with a pillow or cushion!

'Brown-Eye Cowgirl' Relaxation

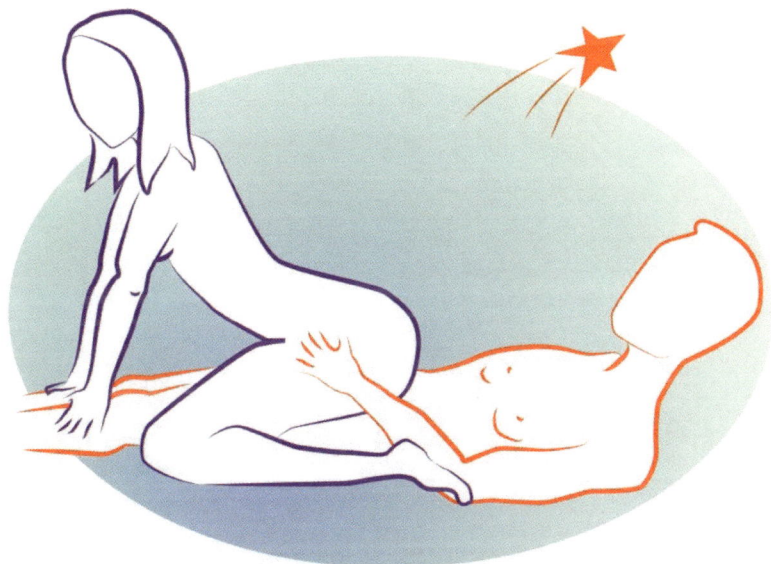

The *'Brown Eye Cowgirl'* is probably one of the most exciting sex positions for the Over 50s. The man lies on his back and the woman she kneels astride her partner but with her back to him as if in the 'Magic Ride', but she leans forward to balance herself on his knees. She can slide up and down supporting her weight with her hands on his knees and he can help by lifting her hips as she moves. In this position the girl can really rotate her hips and control her complete orgasm They can both reach each other's key pleasure zones for a bit of additional stimulating play if they so desire. Ideal for the man to rub the girls' anus with his fingers or insert his thumb deep into her anal passage! Very hot for her!

'Tight Squeeze' Embrace

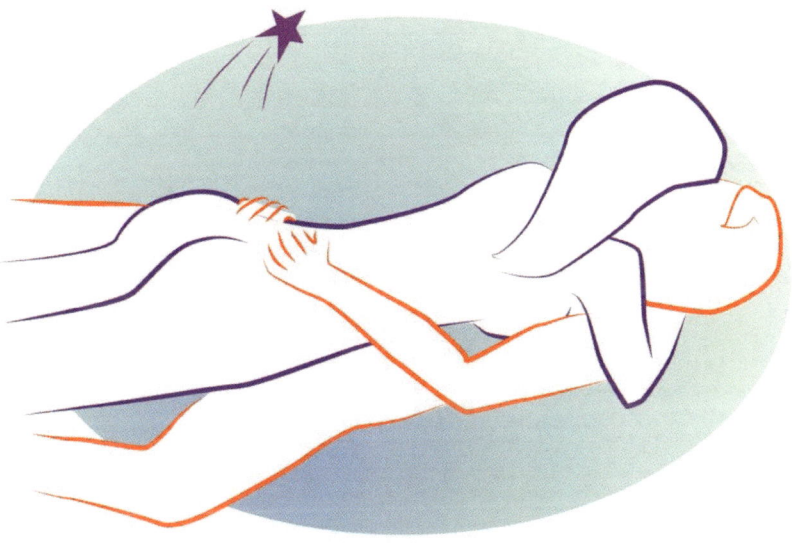

For the *'Tight Squeeze'* she gets her partner to lie down on the bed with his legs stretched out for the very sensual 'Tight Squeeze 'position. She crawls on top of him helping him to enter her. As they come together, she stretches her legs straight out behind her and starts to move back and forth as fast or as slow as she likes. It's a great position for full body contact, kissing and touching throughout. Also a great position for well-endowed man as he won't penetrate her too deeply.

'Straight Coffee Table' Delight

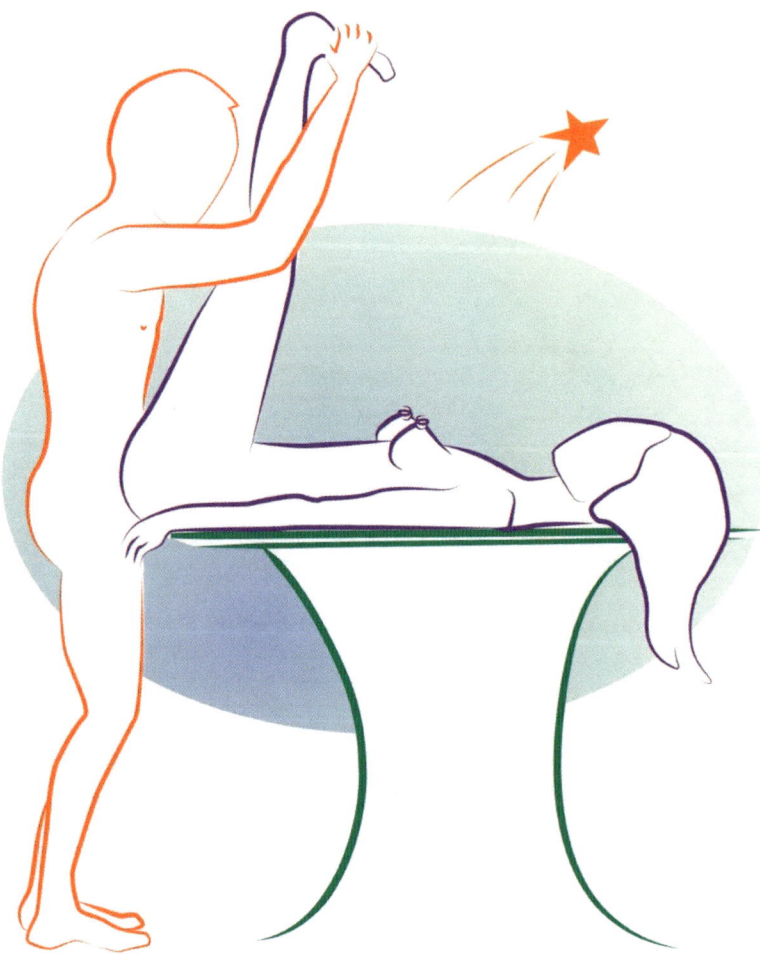

The *'Straight Coffee Table'* position demands certain flexibility!   The woman sits down on a table edge.   The man stands before the table and bends his legs so he's in the best position for immediate penetration.

Now she braces herself by putting her arms around his neck, pulls first the right, then the left leg up onto his shoulders.   She leans back and he directs the thrusting by holding on to her curvaceous bottom!   Just make sure the table is weighted down or secured.

'Presentation' Sensation

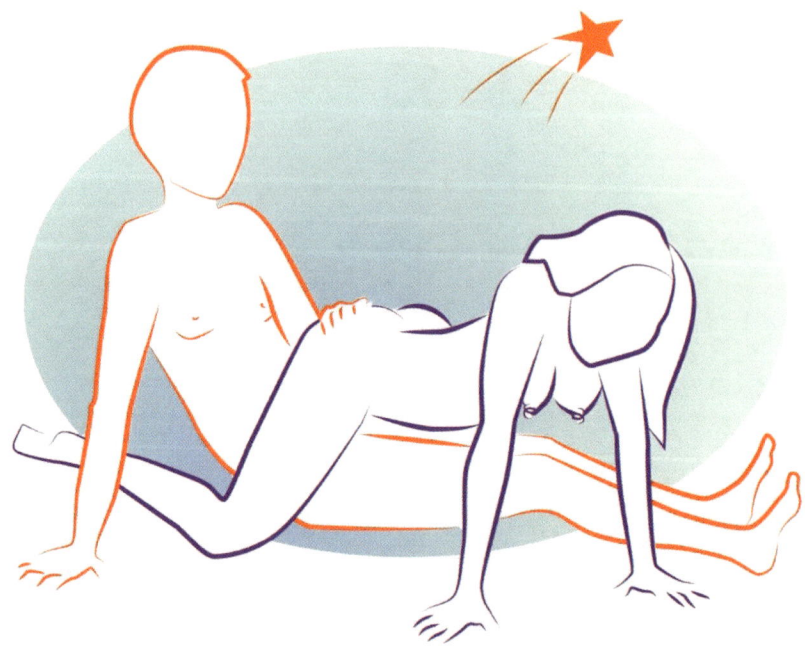

In the *'Presentation'* he is in the sitting position placing his weight on his right arm and his legs outstretched. She sits astride him, with her back to him and leans forwards, supporting herself on her arms. She controls the movement and his hands are free to caress her bottom and could stroke or penetrate her anus if she so desires. Really ideal for anal thumb penetration!

Stretching for Kamasutra

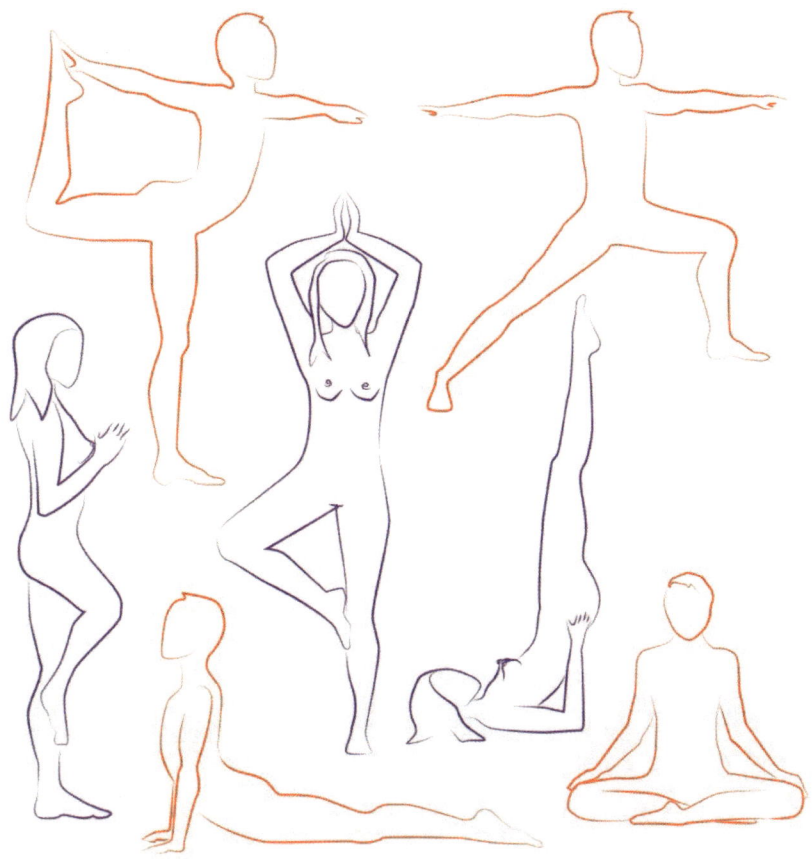

These pre-kamasutra stretch positions are explained in detail below. We selected each possible stretch position so that you and your partner can easily slip into any of our 'Over 50' positions. We strongly recommend you both do these simple exercises naked and together. Considerate it a simple yet erotic warm-up for things to come!

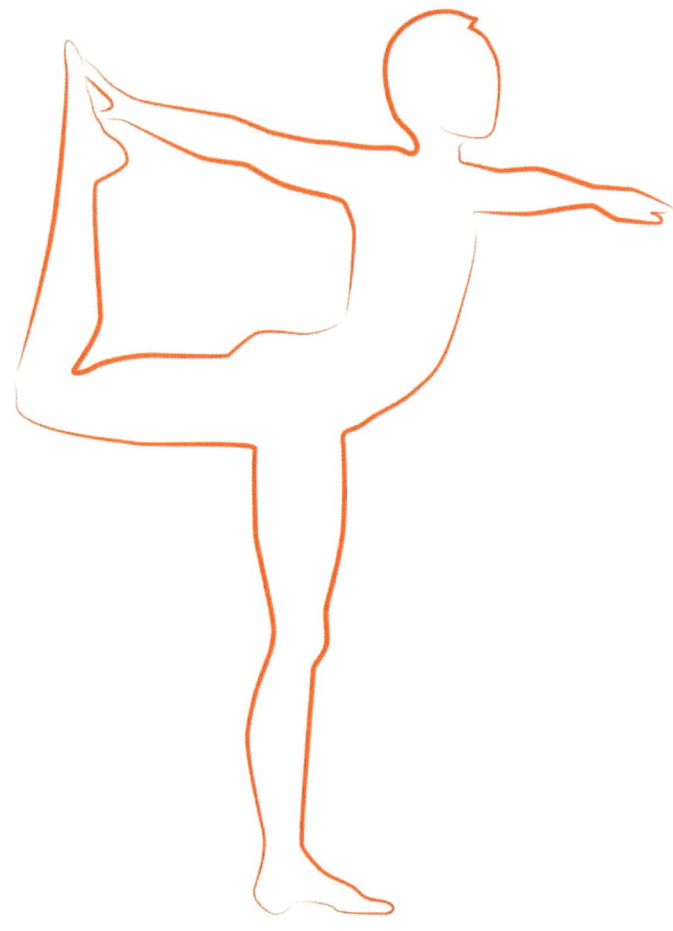

Improve your balance and gently stretch both legs and lower back. Make sure you have no clothes on and your partner is watching! She will just love your style. Take your time get your balance and stretch!

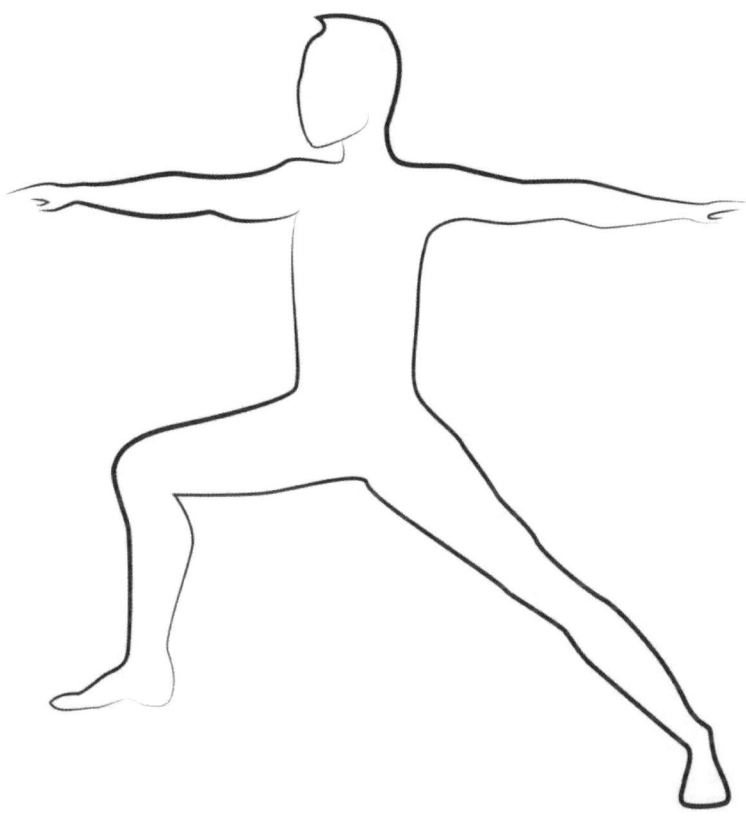

Full exposure 'body stretch'. Great for loosening up those legs, thighs and groin areas whilst giving your partner a full frontal. You may never get past this position if your partner is nearby but persist!

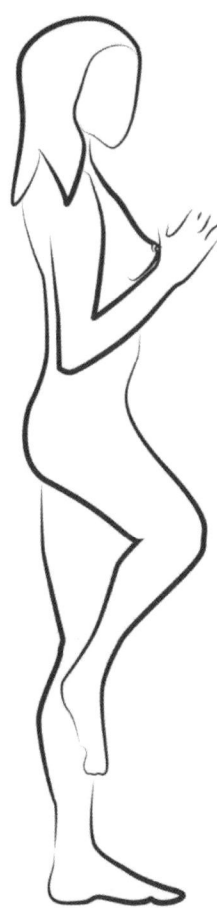

The 'Standing Prayer' position is ideal way to gain balance and poise whilst watching your partner. Very simple calming exercise that focuses your mind on what you intend to do next. Considerate it a spiritual guidance!

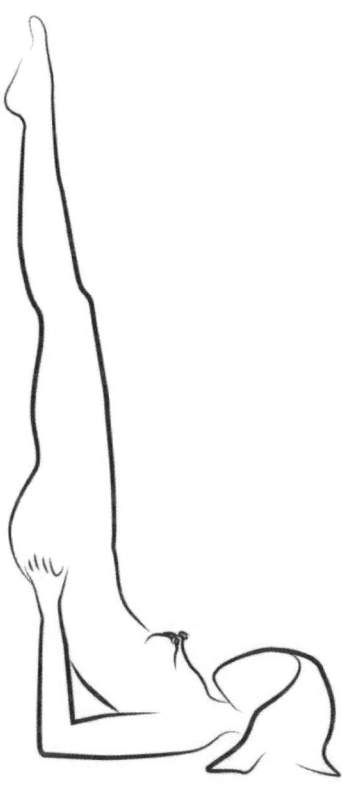

Not easy to do the 'shoulder stand' but great for re-energizing you as the blood flows to your head and gets you thinking naughty thoughts. If you need a help with this position get your partner to support your legs and buttocks. I guarantee you this position will get you instantaneous results.

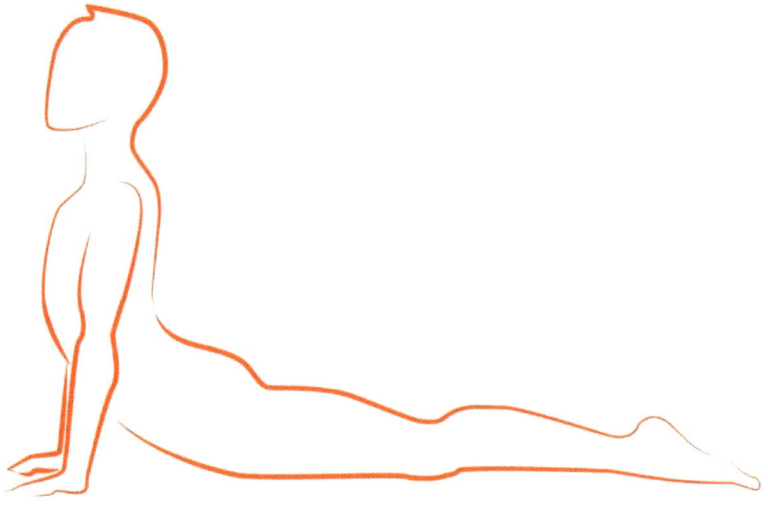

The 'arch' stretch really limbers up your lower back and stretches and strengthens arms and chest. A very erotic position for the lady partner, with her partner observing. Easy to slip directly into many of the Kamasutra positions especially the fondling rider!

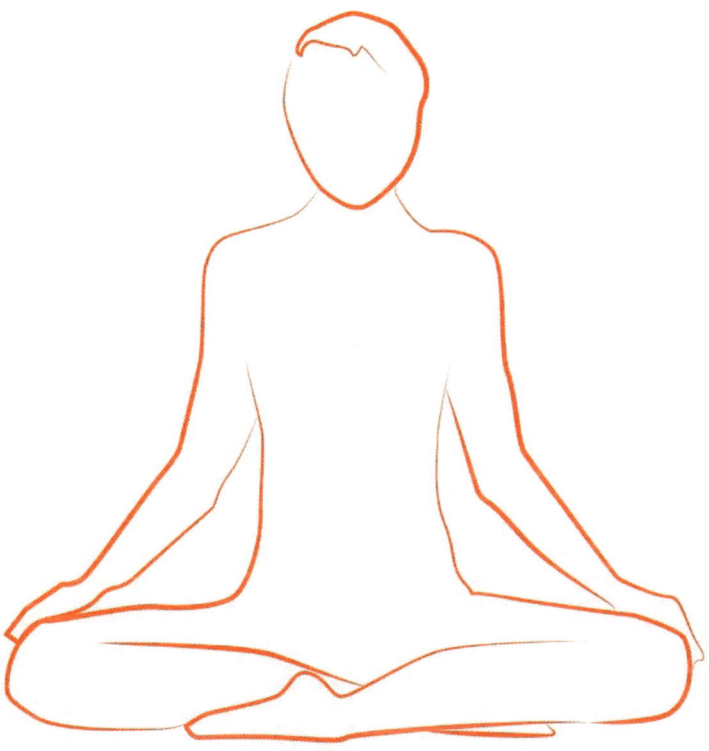

The 'seat' stretch position is fabulous for stretching knees, thighs and groin areas.   A very calming position and a great start for the Kamasutra 'secret whispers'

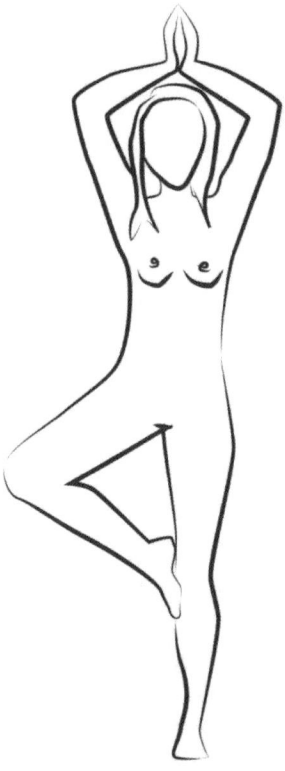

The 'balance' position allows easy stretching of hands, arms and legs whilst giving you poise and balance.   Ideal to do together facing each other.

Now you are ready for the 'Over 50s Kamasutra….Enjoy!

About the Author

Will Thomas McCleat - W.T.   McCleat

Will was born in the Midwest.   Living on a farm growing up, Will was around the farming culture from an early age.   He went to a public school with the farm community values, defining the curriculum; strict immovable subjects that prepared him for the basics in life only.   In his early teens, like many kids in his town he had his first job and first girlfriend.

At twenty-one after graduating from college he was commissioned and reported to flight school.   Receiving his wings eighteen months later he went to a real squadron to learn how to fly a combat airplane.   He soon transitioned to the OV-10A and found himself in Vietnam.   For a small town country boy the assignments took him to exotic parts of the world where he learned not only the art of war but developed a loved of exotic cultures in the variety of countries he was able to visit.   When Will wasn't in the combat zone, he spent his rest and recuperation (R&R) time-off to see as much of the Far East as he could.

In the early 70's, Will's year and a half being in and out of the combat zone, ended his tour because of a disabling wound. He returned to the US to heal and for his final tour of duty. After his years in the military Will was not in any rush to discover his new calling.   He admitted later that his focus was on the love of his life! Will's wealth of experiences and his ability to retain and recall information was something he wanted to communicate to others. He was always fascinated with the why of some things and what if it was not that way? Will decided to build a career as an author and self-publisher so he could express himself in fictional characters.

Will's books are built upon first hand personal experience and about stories he recalled from others. He successfully blends his own experience in novels that can have hot and steamy relationship weaved around true love stories from page one. Will is now a successful writer and has many novels to his name. He lives in what he and the love of his life call their small corner of the world.

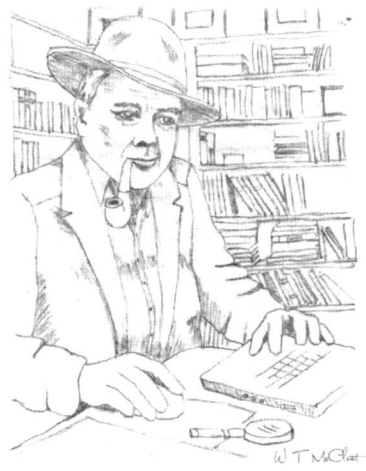

If you liked this book you'd like our book on 'Kamasutra Sex Positions: Sex Positions with Seductive Cocktails' on Amazon in Paperback and on Kindle!

29261846R10053

Made in the USA
Lexington, KY
20 January 2014